Overcoming Infertility

A Woman's Guide to Pregnancy

Gerald M. Honoré, Ph.D., M.D.
Jay S. Nemiro, M.D.

Addicus Books, Inc.
Omaha, Nebraska

An Addicus Nonfiction Book

ISBN 978-1-886039-16-2

Cover design and illustrations by Jack Kusler
Photo of human sperm by Jason Burns/Dr. Ryder/Phototake USA

This book is not intended to serve as a substitute for a physician. Nor is it the authors' intent to give medical advice contrary to that of an attending physician.

Library of Congress Cataloging-in-Publication Data
Honoré, Gerard M., 1957-
   Overcoming infertility : a woman's guide to getting pregnant /
Gerard M. Honoré, Jay S. Nemiro.
      p. Cm.
   Includes index.
   ISBN 978-1-886039-16-2 (alk. Paper)
1. Infertility—Popular works. 2. Infertility—Treatment—Popular
works. I.
   Nemiro, Jay S., 1950- II. Title.
RC889.H53 2010
618.1'78—dc22   2010021381

Addicus Books, Inc.
P.O. Box 45327
Omaha, Nebraska 68145
www.AddicusBooks.com

Printed in the United States of America
10   9   8   7   6   5   4   3   2   1

To my wife, Erika, and my children, Jossie and Wolf,
for putting sunshine in every single day;
and to the memory of my mother, Ellen Stone Honoré Ryan,
for her unfailing love, generosity,
and the riches of opportunity she gave me.
—Gerald M. Honoré, Ph.D., M.D.

To my wonderful wife, Gina—my life partner;
to my six children, whom I thank for their love, patience,
and understanding; to my entire staff, for their loyalty
and commitment to excellence; and to all our patients,
past and present, whose courage, grace,
and strength I continue to admire.
—Jay S. Nemiro, M.D.

Contents

Acknowledgments vii

Introduction ix

1 Infertility: An Overview 1

2 Coping Emotionally 4

3 Female Infertility 12

4 Getting a Diagnosis 26

5 Treatment with Fertility Drugs 42

6 Fertility Treatment Procedures 49

7 Reproductive Surgery 68

8 Male Infertility 72

9 Treatment for Male Infertility 87

10 Donor Sperm 92

11 Donor Eggs and Embryos 98

12 Gestational Carriers 105

Glossary 111

Resources 127

Index 130

About the Authors 141

Acknowledgments

I wish to extend my sincerest thanks to Bob Schenken, M.D., and Jeff Deaton, M.D., for not only being unmatched as teachers, mentors, and friends, but for also being models of personal and professional excellence. They set standards few of us will achieve, but to which we should all aspire.

I also acknowledge Alisa Zinsmeyer Young, M.A., for her invaluable original contributions to this book in the fields of infertility counseling and coping. I am grateful for her professional expertise and for sharing so generously with us and with our readers.

Finally, though no less important, I wish to thank Chris Hinz and Rod Colvin of Addicus Books for their enthusiasm, professional editorial guidance, and lots of plain hard work in every phase of bringing this book to life.

—Gerard M. Honoré, Ph.D., M.D.

I want to thank a number of people who, directly or indirectly, have helped make this book possible. I would like to acknowledge my professors and teachers throughout college and medical school; they guided me through challenging years of hard work and motivated me to stay the course. I thank Richard Falk, M.D., a superb mentor who had enough faith in me to recommend me as Georgetown University's first fellow in reproductive endocrinology and infertility. I acknowledge all the OB/GYN residents who continually challenged me to be a better teacher. I also thank Robert W. McGaughey, Ph.D., whose twenty-four-year partnership as our IVF lab director has helped thousands of our patients to become parents.

I would like to acknowledge my wife, Gina, who has been an ongoing source of inspiration and who continues to be supportive of me in my work, which often requires long days and nights. I am grateful to my six children, Aria, Shane, Talia, Judd, Ashley, and Chad, who are a daily reminder of why I do what I do. I thank my staff, without whom I could not practice the quality of medicine our patients deserve. I extend a very special thank you to all our patients, past and present, who are now the parents of nearly 10,000 babies—miracles of love and science.

Finally, I would like to thank Chris Hinz for her excellent editorial support and Rod Colvin of Addicus Books for his encouragement and for publishing this book on such an important topic.

—Jay S. Nemiro, M.D.

Introduction

In my practice as a reproductive endocrinologist, I've met thousands of women who have tried, without success, to have a baby of their own. I have seen firsthand the emotional distress these women endure, and I understand how these feelings can cast dark shadows on every part of their lives. My goal is to help these women become mothers. First, we must find the "road" to take to accomplish that goal. I begin by asking questions in effort to discover why she is not getting pregnant. Once I have more information, we can start drawing out the map—the plan for reaching a diagnosis and the plan for treatment.

When I first meet a woman in my office, we begin the first of many important conversations. I always try to listen carefully to her concerns and share with her as much information as she seeks. I believe real knowledge can give peace of mind, and that knowledge along with emotional support brings inner strength. It is the treatment plan and this strength that takes these women and their partners to eventual success.

I hope this book serves as a resource that gives these many brave women the answers to their important questions. My goal with the book is provide readers with the knowledge, strength, and hope they need to take their journeys toward families of their own.

— Gerard M. Honoré, Ph.D., M.D.

My intention in writing this book is to make the journey a little less stressful for women who are trying to have a child. I hope this book will empower you and your partner by giving you useful information. Having had the privilege of working with thousands of couples who have faced infertility, I've found that knowledge leads to understanding, and understanding leads to empowerment.

By knowing how infertility can occur and the challenges it can pose for both you and your partner, you'll be better equipped to make informed decisions about issues ranging from diagnostic tests to treatment. You'll also be ready to handle the emotional and psychological roller coaster that often accompanies each development and decision throughout fertility treatment.

I encourage you to find a physician with whom you can develop a true partnership—a doctor who is committed to providing competent, compassionate care and who also understands the fears and feelings a woman may experience in attempting to achieve her dream of becoming a mother. Remember, even if you are successful in getting pregnant, your emotional journey continues. You'll want the continued support of your physician.

It is my hope that, once you have a healthy baby in your arms, you will be able to relax and enjoy motherhood, and you will look back and say it was all worth it.

—Jay S. Nemiro, M.D.

1

Infertility: An Overview

Not being able to have a baby can be heartbreaking. You no doubt know the frustration. Perhaps you grew up believing that one day you'd be a mother. Now you're not so certain. You're also not alone. It's estimated that as many as 10 percent of reproductive-age females are grappling with *infertility*, the inability to conceive after one year of unprotected intercourse.

However, just because you haven't conceived doesn't mean you can't. Infertility is a medical problem that can be diagnosed and treated much as any other health issue. Over the past few decades, medical science has made great strides in treating both female and male infertility. So you needn't lose hope. With help, it's quite possible that you *can* have a baby.

Infertility: A Shared Problem

As a woman, you may feel solely responsible for your inability to conceive. However, infertility is not just a female problem. In fact, nearly 40 to 50 percent of infertility cases involve factors related to the male. In 10 to 35 percent of cases, both the female and the male have a fertility problem. Another 15 to 20 percent of cases are said to be unexplained—meaning doctors don't have a concrete reason for a couple's inability to conceive.

Common Causes of Infertility

In women, the most common causes of infertility involve ovulation factors and a diminishing supply of quality eggs. Most women ovulate normally into their late twenties; however, by age thirty-five to thirty-eight, the ability to ovulate normally may decline. Ovulation may also be affected by factors such as thyroid problems and hormone imbalances. Other major causes of female infertility involve problems with the fallopian tubes, cervix, and/or uterus.

In men, the focus is on the quantity and quality of sperm. Age is not usually a factor in a man's ability to produce sperm; however, any damage to his reproductive organs can cause problems with sperm production and delivery.

In addition, certain lifestyle factors may affect the ability of both sexes to conceive. For example, in women, Chlamydia infections and other sexually transmitted diseases (STDs) can damage the fallopian tubes, resulting in infertility. In men, the use of alcohol, marijuana, and other recreational drugs has well-documented harmful effects on sperm production.

Smoking tobacco may or may not be harmful to reproduction. Some studies show that nicotine and other chemicals from smoking can impair the ovaries and interfere with their ability to create *estradiol*, the hormone specifically involved in egg production. In fact, some estimates are that tobacco use reduces fertility in both females and males by about 15 percent. Other research, however, shows no evidence of this effect.

Keep in mind that couples aren't tested for infertility simply because they drink alcohol or smoke. They're screened for infertility because they've been unsuccessful in their pregnancy attempts. Previous behaviors may come up in the evaluation, but there are likely other reasons for the problem.

Types of Infertility

Couples who have never conceived are said to have *primary infertility*. Couples who are unable to conceive even though they've had a child previously have *secondary infertility*. In fact, infertility sometimes first surfaces when a couple attempts to have a second child. In many cases, however, couples experience both primary and secondary infertility.

Treatment for Infertility

Thanks to modern technology, help is available for couples having difficulty conceiving. The treatments, described later in this book, range from fertility drugs that can help the ovaries release eggs to microsurgery that can repair physical problems in both women and men. The biggest treatment breakthrough in reproductive technology during the past thirty years has been *in vitro fertilization* (*IVF*), a procedure in which fertilization occurs outside the body when an egg and sperm are joined in a laboratory; the embryo is then implanted in the woman's uterus.

Costs for Treatment

The costs linked to fertility treatment can vary greatly, depending on the procedures you have done, where you live, and which doctor you see. Treatment costs can run into tens of thousands of dollars if you and your partner must undergo high-tech procedures, use donor eggs, or engage a gestational carrier.

Does Insurance Pay?

Although infertility is considered a disease, insurance coverage for fertility treatment is mandated in fewer than fifteen states. That means there's a good chance you'll be paying out-of-pocket for most of your treatment.

Even if your insurer offers coverage, there's wide variance in which services are covered. For example, an IVF procedure may be specifically excluded, or it may be included only if you use your own eggs and your partner's sperm. In other cases, your policy might require that you have a specific history of infertility resulting from a condition considered to be a general health problem, such as endometriosis or fibroid tumors. In addition, your policy might require that you be under a certain age, or it may have a lifetime limit covering a maximum number of treatment cycles for each covered procedure.

If you see a fertility specialist, someone in his or her office will discuss costs and your insurance coverage with you. It's important to understand the costs early on, so that you don't encounter additional stress due to unexpected financial obligations.

2

Coping Emotionally

Not being able to get pregnant when you want a child can be a painful and isolating experience. As you worry about whether you'll ever become a mother, it may seem as if women all around you are having babies. You may feel that most people don't understand what you're going through emotionally—your longing to be pregnant, to experience childbirth, and to bond with an infant. Indeed, it hurts deeply, and the despair can take a toll on your self-esteem. So how do you overcome the disappointment and navigate the frustrations? By marshaling your inner reserve and gaining support from your partner and others around you, you can cope with infertility.

Understand the Challenges

To cope emotionally—and to keep your relationship with your partner intact—it's important that you understand the emotional challenges ahead of you. Not surprisingly, infertility evokes many of the same feelings that people experience with the death of a loved one—denial...anger...guilt...blame... depression...and acceptance. Of course, mourning your hopes and dreams is different from mourning the loss of a loved one; nonetheless, the emotions can be quite similar.

Denial

Many couples try to get pregnant on their own for years before they finally seek help. Filled with hope, they keep trying, believing that they'll eventually conceive. However, denying that a problem may exist only serves to intensify your disappointment and delay potentially helpful treatment.

Anger

Being angry is a normal emotional response to infertility. It is simply an outward sign of frustration over not being in control of events and the emotions those events evoke. The more you understand your anger, the more likely you are to express it in an appropriate manner—and not in ways that are destructive to you or the people around you.

Guilt and Blame

When you're searching for answers, it's natural to wonder if you did something in the past to cause your infertility. But dwelling on the past can sap your energy and prevent you from moving forward. If the blame is directed toward your partner, it can lead to a breakdown in your relationship at a time when you need each other the most.

Depression

When you grieve, it's also normal to become depressed. However, with time and emotional support, you can bounce back. But if you exhibit any signs of severe or clinical depression—apathy, intense anxiety, fatigue, poor concentration, or the inability to make decisions—you may need professional help. Fortunately, many counselors specialize in infertility counseling. Antidepressants can also help lift depression.

Gather Your Coping Skills

Seeking help for your infertility is usually a sign that you've accepted the fact that something is wrong and you need to find answers. It's a positive first step. That doesn't mean that you won't experience disappointment or doubt as you're being evaluated and treated. You may face multiple procedures before you experience success, and you'll likely still wonder at times if you'll ever conceive or carry a baby to full term. But hearing that your infertility actually has a medical cause—and, more than likely, some treatment options—will alleviate much of your distress. What else can you do? No matter where you are in the fertility treatment process, there are simple steps you can take to stay focused, energized, and emotionally healthy.

Be Informed

Understanding your problem—and leaving the guesswork behind—is essential to coping. Being informed will help you to understand the medical tests and treatments being recommended, allowing you to weigh the risks against the rewards. The more you learn, the more empowered you'll feel.

Keep Your Options Open

You'll probably have a very clear idea of your goals when you begin the fertility treatment process. But as realities change, you may need to reassess your options. What once seemed like an unacceptable choice may become the preferable alternative. Your doctor will likely outline the treatment alternatives in the beginning, focusing on the best probability for success. Then, if a therapy doesn't work in a reasonable amount of time, you'll need to decide on the next step. Try to stay flexible.

Manage Your Stress

No matter how hard you try, it's unlikely that you can eliminate all your anxieties about your infertility and the treatment process. It's not uncommon to feel apprehension, nervousness, and even panic, but there are things you can do to manage those feelings.

Eat right, exercise daily, and get sufficient sleep. A nutritious diet and a good exercise program can empower you physically and emotionally. Sleep loss is emotionally debilitating, so get plenty of rest.

Join a support group. Communicating with others who are grappling with infertility can be most helpful. Participating in a support group can ease the sense of isolation and help lift depression. Organizations such as RESOLVE, the National Infertility Association (www.resolve.org), host support groups throughout the country. Your fertility clinic may also sponsor group sessions.

Keep a "gratitude" journal. Journaling is an effective way to express your emotions and chronicle your progress. Some women find it helpful to journal affirmations to themselves— positive things in the midst of the tension and anxiety.

Practice meditation and yoga. By channeling your thoughts and disciplining your body, you can relieve stress.

Keep Your Infertility in Perspective

It's easy to let "having a baby" become the focus of your entire life. But try to avoid letting it dominate your conversations or, for that matter, your daily life. Maintaining a normal routine during fertility treatment may seem challenging at times. Couples often plan their activities around their infertility procedures. Or they avoid situations that remind them that they don't have the family they want. But allowing your infertility to dominate your thinking isolates you emotionally. Instead, try to do things you'd usually do and see people you'd normally see.

Get Support from Your Partner

When it comes to emotional support, you need it first from your partner. But since infertility evokes so many passions and expectations, your mate may not always give you what you need. Your partner may want to be loyal, caring, and sympathetic, but may say and do the "wrong" things. How do you get the support you need? There are steps you can take to ensure that you feel supported by your partner and that your relationship survives the infertility experience.

Understand Your Partner's Anxieties

As a woman, you're dealing with your own particular anxieties—but remember, your partner is likely dealing with many of his own. On the one hand, he may be concerned for you if you're the one undergoing the tests and procedures. He may feel like a helpless bystander. On the other hand, he may be stressed by his own role, especially if his sperm is deemed inadequate. No matter how much you reassure him that his sperm count is not a measure of his manhood, he may feel guilty and ashamed. Men often believe that their masculinity is diminished if their partner can't get pregnant.

In addition, you and your partner may have entirely different coping mechanisms. Your partner's silence may mask his pain, while you may feel relieved when you express your emotions. By understanding your differences and making allowances for them, you'll improve your communication.

Ask for What You Need

As close as you and your partner may be, you can't expect him to read your mind. Even in the best relationships, people need to make clear what they need. Many times, you may simply need to have your partner listen to you and acknowledge that he understands what you're going through.

You may feel supported by having your partner attend fertility evaluations and treatments with you. If so, ask him to attend as many appointments as possible. (Many men don't attend if they're not asked.) By being actively involved in the process, your partner will learn more and will likely be more understanding of what you're going through.

Protect Your Relationship

Failing to conceive is often the first crisis a couple faces together. And the fertility treatment process—particularly if it's long, complicated, or painful—can add to the strain. The good news is that most couples survive; some even become stronger. Unfortunately, for others, the stress ultimately ends the relationship. Perhaps one partner wants children more than the other partner does. The difference may not be immediately apparent, but if the stress builds, it can produce a flash point. One partner may demand an end to the treatment, while the other wants to continue.

Of course, if you and your partner disagree on the fundamentals of your relationship, you may have issues beyond just having a baby. But if the problems you're experiencing with infertility involve a lack of communication or mounting stress, you can find ways to overcome those issues. For instance, by scheduling time each day to discuss infertility issues, you allow yourselves the opportunity to express your feelings and concerns, but free up the remaining hours to talk about other things. It's important that you be honest with each other and focus on understanding what each of you is feeling.

Many couples complain that their sex life is no longer spontaneous or enjoyable because it has become centered on conception. Other factors may also affect sexual intimacy during fertility treatment. For example, some medications and procedures increase the size of a woman's ovaries, making intercourse physically uncomfortable for her. At some points in treatment, a couple may even be asked to avoid sex completely.

It's important to realize that your sex life will be spontaneous and enjoyable again. In the meantime, by taking advantage of the quality time you do have together and finding ways to cement your relationship beyond sexual intimacy, you can actually enrich your relationship. Remember that you were a loving couple before you wanted to be parents. Perhaps it's time to rekindle that spark that first brought you together.

Get Support from Your Family and Friends

Telling other people about your infertility can be stressful. For most couples, infertility is a very private and emotionally charged topic. It can be even more painful to discuss if you sense that others don't understand what you're feeling. Perhaps you'll choose to keep such personal information to yourself. Yet bringing others into your confidence and asking for their support can be a healthy step in coping with infertility.

How do you identify confidants? Deciding who to tell and what to tell can be difficult. Rely on your intuition, and reach out to family members and friends you know you can trust and who you know will understand. There may be others whom you feel you *need* to inform—your supervisor, for example, if you'll need time off from work. On the other hand, you may not feel the need to share details with co-workers and casual acquaintances.

Set Emotional Boundaries

You can also protect yourself emotionally by setting emotional boundaries. For example, it's important to let your confidants know how best to lend their support. Not everyone will be as educated as you've become about infertility, so it may help to provide your confidants with basic information on what you're going through. Since the process can have many highs and lows, you may need different things from them at different times. You may want advice if you're at a crossroads. You may need empathy when you want to cry. Or you may want to share your joy when you become pregnant. By communicating specifically what you need, you help those around you respond appropriately.

Being around people who have babies may evoke feelings of sadness and envy. You may find that you're uncomfortable attending events such as baby showers or gatherings with new parents. You don't have to attend. As long as you're not isolating yourself, it's okay to decline some invitations.

Plan Your Responses

Knowing how to respond to the unsolicited remarks and advice of others is an empowering tool. Perhaps you've heard your share of "What, you're not pregnant yet?" or "You just need to relax, and it will happen." Even though people mean well, their comments can be frustrating.

It may be easy to dismiss the comments of casual acquaintances since you may not feel the need to disclose personal information, but when your parents, siblings, or closest friends ask what seem to be insensitive questions, it hurts. How do you handle these situations? First, recognize that they care about you and may simply be "clumsy" with the topic. Perhaps then you can acknowledge that you know they love you and reassure them that you're working on the matter. If you're comfortable doing so, you can even share details of your treatment with them.

Ending Treatment

There may come a time when you need to decide if it's best to stop treatment. Understandably, this is a difficult decision to make. How can you tell when it's time to change course? It may be time when:

- your preoccupation with getting pregnant is interfering with your life, including your relationships with your partner and others
- you've tried all the treatments you had planned to try
- you're physically and emotionally exhausted
- you're feeling the strain of debt incurred to pay for treatments

Although there are often practical reasons to end treatment, your instincts will likely tell you when it's time to stop. You will know in your heart that it's time to move on. That knowledge may be painful, but remind yourself that you have investigated the potential problems and tried many promising treatments.

Most physicians suggest taking a six-month break from treatment to confirm your feelings. If you're confident in your decision, you'll have a sense of closure. You'll feel you're not quitting, but making a choice to stop. You may even look forward to opening new doors on the rest of your life. Later, if your intuition tells you to go on, you can explore any remaining treatment options.

3

Female Infertility

pproximately 50 percent of conception difficulties involve female factors. Under normal circumstances, your body orchestrates the process of ovulation and conception with fine-tuned precision. However, many factors can impede your ability to conceive and carry a baby to full term. To better understand those factors, let's first review how the female reproductive system works. You'll have a better appreciation of what your doctor might want to investigate.

The Basics of Female Reproduction

The female reproductive system is a complex one involving organs, glands, and hormones. If you are being tested for infertility, your doctor will likely perform a physical examination of your *ovaries, fallopian tubes, uterus, cervix,* and vagina. He or she will also order blood tests to check your hormone function.

Ovaries

These olive-shaped glands are located on each side of the uterus. Typically, every month, one of them releases a mature egg, accompanied by *estrogen* and *progesterone*, hormones that promote uterine lining changes necessary for pregnancy. If fertilization doesn't occur, the lining and egg are lost through menstruation.

Fallopian Tubes

Pregnancy actually begins in one of the two trumpet-shaped fallopian tubes linking your ovaries and uterus. During ovulation, one tube's feathery projections capture a mature egg, which then slowly moves toward the uterus, hopefully linking with sperm along the way. Once the egg and sperm unite in the tube, the resulting embryo is ushered into the uterus.

Uterus

Comprised largely of muscle, the uterus supports and nourishes a growing fetus. When you're not pregnant, your uterus is the size and shape of a small pear. During pregnancy, the cavity expands to hold a full-term baby. The lining of the uterus—called the *endometrium*—thickens every month in anticipation of an embryo. If pregnancy doesn't occur, the lining breaks down and sheds in your menstrual flow.

Cervix

The cervix is a small, circular muscle separating the uterus from the vagina. During most of your menstrual cycle, cervical mucus acts as a barrier to the uterus. But prior to ovulation, the mucus transforms into a watery substance that invites sperm. With pregnancy, the cervix first lengthens to hold the fetus, then shortens for labor, and finally expands to accommodate delivery.

Vagina

Extending from the *vulva*, or external folds of the genitalia, to the cervical opening, or neck, of the uterus, the vagina is a muscular canal that stretches to accommodate the penis. During sexual arousal, the vagina's vessel-rich walls fill with blood, while the two small glands at its entrance—the *Bartholin glands*—secrete fluids that lubricate the space.

Hormones

Your reproductive organs may be ready and able, but you can't get pregnant unless they work with precision. Hormones orchestrate your menstrual cycle. In addition to the ovaries, which produce several types of estrogen and progesterone, the other hormone-control centers are the *hypothalamus* and the

Female Reproductive System

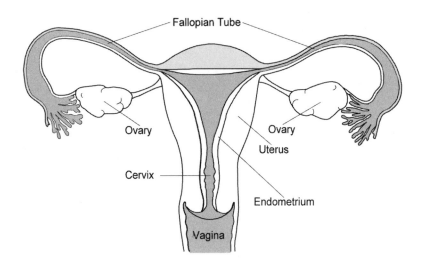

Fallopian Tube

Ovary

Ovary

Uterus

Cervix

Endometrium

Vagina

pituitary gland. (The role of hormones is discussed further in chapter 4.)

Hypothalamus

This cherry-size gland located in the midbrain regulates the nervous and endocrine systems. By sending chemical messengers, such as *gonadotropin-releasing hormone (GnRH)*, to the pituitary gland, the hypothalamus starts a cascade of events that sparks your sexual response, tells your ovaries when to produce eggs, and prepares your uterus and cervix for pregnancy.

Pituitary Gland

About the size of a pea, this gland "answers" the hypothalamus by releasing *follicle-stimulating hormone (FSH)* and *luteinizing hormone (LH)*. FSH signals eggs to mature within individual ovarian *follicles;* LH triggers the release of one randomly selected egg with the potential to be fertilized.

Phases of the Menstrual Cycle

Your menstrual cycle is the framework in which your hormones drive your reproductive organs to do their work. With a typical cycle, each month between puberty and menopause, a woman's body prepares for the possibility of pregnancy. The length of the menstrual cycle varies from woman to woman and from month to month, but the average cycle is twenty-eight days. A good rule of thumb is that if your cycle is between twenty-five and thirty-three days, you're within the normal range. If it's absent, chronically irregular, or falls outside those margins, you're likely not ovulating on a regular basis.

The rise and fall of your hormones affect three distinct phases of your cycle.

The follicular phase. Extending from the first day of your menstrual period to ovulation, the follicular phase is when the egg-bearing follicles in your ovaries develop. Your pituitary gland is increasing its secretion of FSH to spur the growth of ten to fifteen fluid-filled follicles, or sacs, each containing a single egg. Typically, one egg will become dominant and eventually be released. (Although most women release only one egg per month, some have the genetic tendency to release two or more eggs, resulting in natural twins [1 in 90], triplets [1 in 8,100], or quadruplets [1 in 729,000].) The follicular phase is sometimes referred to as the *proliferative phase* in reference to the endometrium, because while the old lining is shedding, a new one is growing in anticipation of conception next month.

The ovulatory phase. Although the egg finally bursts from its follicle during this stage, the timing is hardly precise. Normal ovulation occurs fourteen days before the onset of your next menstrual period, which, in a perfect twenty-eight-day cycle, also means day fourteen. But even within a normal cycle, ovulation can occur anytime between days twelve and sixteen. If your cycle is longer than twenty-eight days, it might even occur as late as day eighteen. In any case, ovulation is always prefaced by a surge of the pituitary hormone LH; the surge occurs twenty-six to forty hours prior to release of the egg.

Since egg selection seems to be random, there's no way to determine which ovary will release the egg each month; on average, though, this alternates in most women. No matter which ovary is involved, the selected dominant egg, once released, begins its slow descent into your fallopian tube, a nourishing environment where fertilization takes place.

The luteal phase. Once the egg is released, the leftover follicle reorganizes into a structure called the *corpus luteum.* The corpus luteum secretes increasing amounts of progesterone, which, together with estrogen, causes the uterine lining to double in thickness. If you conceive, the embryo floats in the uterus for several days before implanting in the lining in order to grow.

If conception occurs, *human chorionic gonadotropin* (*hCG*), considered the hormone of pregnancy, continues to stimulate the corpus luteum to produce progesterone until the placenta is fully functional and can produce its own hormones. This step generally occurs at the end of the first *trimester,* or beginning of the thirteenth week. If conception does not occur, the corpus luteum degenerates and is eventually reabsorbed by the ovary. With no estrogen and progesterone production, the uterus sheds its lining, starting menstruation.

Causes of Female Infertility

Ovulatory Factors

The most common cause of female infertility, ovulatory problems represent about 25 to 30 percent of all cases. Even if your reproductive organs are structurally and functionally sound, pregnancy cannot occur unless you produce a healthy egg, capable of being fertilized. Your ability to produce a healthy egg is entirely dependent on good ovarian function. In order for your ovaries to produce eggs that mature and release, the five major hormones that drive your menstrual cycle—estradiol (a form of estrogen), progesterone, GnRH, FSH, and LH—need to be functioning normally.

If your cycle differs from what's considered normal, it may indicate a problem with ovulation. For example, if your cycle is shorter than twenty-one days or longer than thirty-eight days, you may be *anovulatory,* meaning that you're not ovulating. On the other hand, if your cycle is irregular—occurring at unpredictable intervals—you may be *oligo-ovulatory,* or ovulating occasionally. However, even if your cycle length is normal and you never miss a monthly period, you may still have a problem that impedes your production of eggs. In fact, 3 percent of women have regular cycles but do not release eggs regularly.

What causes such irregularities? As mentioned above, any imbalance of the major hormones involved can disrupt your cycle. Your cycle can also be disrupted if your thyroid or adrenal glands aren't working normally or if your pituitary gland is producing a higher-than-normal level of the hormone *prolactin.* Prolactin stimulates the production of breast milk, but at higher levels in women who are not pregnant or nursing, it can interfere with ovarian function. Your cycle may become irregular, and/or the luteal phase, which normally is the final two weeks, might be too short to create a receptive uterine environment. Any underlying physical problem or circumstance that interferes with your monthly cycle can cause ovulatory disorders or dysfunction, as well. These include:

- physical, emotional, or psychological stress
- excessive exercise
- very low body weight
- obesity (25 percent over ideal body weight)

Most women with ovulatory problems can be helped with medication. As long as you're not menopausal or experiencing *premature ovarian failure (POF),* your doctor likely can regulate your cycle, using a variety of oral or injectable fertility drugs, so that you generate healthy eggs.

Polycystic ovarian syndrome (PCOS). A hormone disorder, polycystic ovarian syndrome (PCOS) is one of the most common ovulatory problems associated with infertility. The syndrome is named for small cysts that form on the ovaries. It occurs in one out of ten women of childbearing age. In addition to infrequent or absent periods, PCOS sufferers usually experience symptoms such as excess facial and body hair, weight gain, and elevated insulin levels, which create a risk for type 2 diabetes.

To diagnose PCOS, your doctor will take your medical history (the syndrome can be hereditary) and perform a pelvic ultrasound and laboratory tests. By first targeting your symptoms with medication, such as insulin-altering drugs, and then regulating your cycle with fertility drugs, your doctor can control your PCOS and put you on the path to pregnancy.

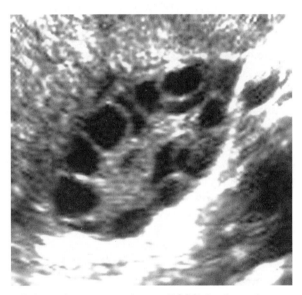

Polycystic ovary syndrome (PCOS) is shown here. The cysts in this ovary ultrasound show up as a ring of black dots.

Age and ovarian reserve. As you get older, you have fewer and fewer viable eggs available for conception; in fact, you have fewer eggs overall. Interestingly, you're born with all the eggs you'll ever have—about 1 million. By your first menstrual cycle, your ovarian reserve will have naturally dwindled to four hundred thousand eggs, a number that will decrease every month until menopause, when you'll have none. (For every one egg you release each month, you lose one thousand.) This natural decline can begin as early as your mid- to late thirties.

Premature ovarian failure (POF). Premature ovarian failure (POF) is defined as loss of normal ovarian function before age forty. This failure results in a greatly diminished reserve of quality eggs and estrogen deficiency, which causes many of the same symptoms as menopause. Because of the similarities, POF is sometimes referred to as premature menopause. But there is a difference. A patient diagnosed with POF can still have sporadic periods and maybe even get pregnant, while someone who's prematurely menopausal usually ceases to have periods.

POF can be triggered by such things as surgery and cancer treatment. Diagnosis of POF is made based on a medical history along with laboratory and imaging tests. Since there's no treatment to restore normal ovarian function, women with POF usually can't get pregnant naturally and must consider donor eggs or adoption.

Tubal Factors

Disorders of the fallopian tubes are the second most common cause of female infertility, accounting for 15 to 20 percent of cases. Tubal disorders can involve a range of problems, from microscopic damage to major dysfunction. Your tubes are a complex neuromuscular system designed to pick up an egg from your ovary, facilitate fertilization, and transport the resulting embryo to your uterus for implantation. When the fallopian tubes are blocked or unable to move, they become a major impediment to conception.

A tube can be fully blocked or technically open but constricted by a partial blockage. Such blockages are usually caused by scarring within the tubes, resulting from surgery, trauma, or infection in the area. Even if a tube is completely open, however, it may not be able to move and pick up an egg because *pelvic adhesions* are holding it in place. These fibrous bands of scar tissue can form in and around your organs, again as a complication of surgery, trauma, or infection in the pelvic region. Some bacterial infections can result in more serious tubal scarring and adhesions known as *pelvic inflammatory disease* (*PID*). Women who've suffered postpartum and other pelvic infections, such as those associated with a ruptured appendix, are at risk for PID.

The biggest bacterial offenders, however, are usually sexually transmitted diseases (STDs). Chlamydia infection, in particular, is an increasingly worrisome medical issue. Unfortunately, 50 percent of women exposed to Chlamydia infection don't know they contracted it. Left untreated, Chlamydia infection can cause serious damage to the fallopian tubes and reproductive organs; it can result in extensive scar tissue and adhesions throughout the pelvic cavity. In fact, every Chlamydia exposure gives you a 25 percent risk of developing tubal disorders. If diagnosed early, however, the infection can be treated successfully with antibiotics, so it's less likely to threaten conception. (Your partner should be treated, too.) If the infection has caused fallopian tube blockages or pelvic adhesions, your doctor will address those problems separately.

Anytime a woman has tubal damage, she's at greater risk for *ectopic pregnancy,* a potentially serious condition in which an embryo implants outside the uterus, usually inside a fallopian tube. If discovered early, the ectopic pregnancy may be dissolved with a chemotherapy agent, methotrexate, before it causes irreparable harm. But if it goes undetected, it can rupture the tube, causing life-threatening bleeding. A doctor will immediately perform surgery to remove the ectopic pregnancy and hope to save the fallopian tube.

Uterine Factors

Uterine problems, which account for about 5 percent of all female infertility cases, include growths and other anomalies in the uterus that make it difficult for an embryo to implant and develop.

Uterine fibroids. Fibroids are slow-growing, benign tumors that develop in the smooth muscle of the uterine wall. They can remain within the uterus or grow outward into the lower pelvic or abdominal area. Studies suggest that as many as 40 percent of women of childbearing age will develop at least one fibroid. Fibroids are more common in African-American women, who have has much as a 50 percent risk of developing one.

Although many women have fibroids, not all women have difficulty with them. Depending on their type, size, and location, these growths may or may not cause the characteristic symptoms of pelvic pain, heavy menstrual bleeding, and bowel or bladder problems. They also may or may not have an impact on your ability to get pregnant and carry a baby to full term. The fibroids that concern fertility specialists the most are *intramural fibroids*, because they develop within the muscular wall of the uterus and can distort the uterine cavity, possibly interfering with conception and causing repeated miscarriages. Also of concern are *submucosal fibroids*, because they can grow through the inside wall lining, shrinking the size of the cavity and making it too small for a growing fetus. Again, they can cause implantation problems or miscarriages.

No matter where they surface, very large fibroids (5 cm or two inches or greater) can be a major problem because they siphon blood away from a developing fetus. Even if the tumors aren't near the baby, they can reroute the flow of nutrients away from the endometrium. They also can "trick" the uterus into thinking it's bigger than it is, resulting in preterm labor or a premature delivery.

Endometrial polyps. Endometrial polyps are fleshy growths that also can interfere with fertility. But they develop from the uterine lining, rather than from the muscle. These polyps can range from tiny to very large in size. The bigger they are, the more they distort the uterine cavity and intrude on conception or pregnancy.

Endometrial polyps don't necessarily grow during pregnancy, but they can become more vascular (blood-filled) and, as a result, bleed easily at critical times, disrupting implantation or increasing the risk of miscarriage. In some cases, polyps need to be surgically removed; in other cases, they don't need treatment. Your doctor will consider the size of each growth and the risks and benefits of removing it.

Other uterine anomalies. A woman's fertility can be impeded by other uterine anomalies, some caused by previous gynecologic procedures, such as *dilation and curettage (D & C)*. This procedure is often performed to investigate abnormal bleeding and other gynecologic problems. Women who have had a D & C sometimes develop *Asherman's syndrome,* a condition in which the walls of the uterus are so scarred from crisscrossing adhesions that they stick together. (Asherman's is also linked to abortions and pelvic inflammatory disease.) There

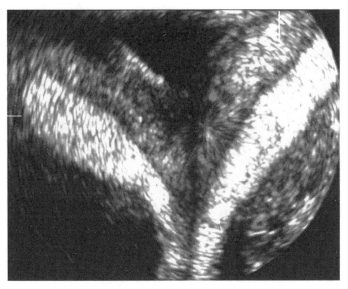

This ultrasound shows a bicornuate uterus, or so-called "heart-shaped" uterus. It can be repaired surgically.

can also be structural anomalies, although not all of them cause problems with fertility. For instance, 20 percent of women have a *retroverted* uterus—one that is tipped backward rather than positioned forward—but this anomaly doesn't impede conception. However, an abnormally shaped uterus, which occurs in 2 to 3 percent of women, can cause difficulties. The major problems occur with the following:

- *Septate uterus.* This abnormal shape—the most common—is caused by a *uterine septum,* a fibrous band that divides the cavity. The septum forms during a woman's own prenatal development. Women with a septum are at risk for miscarriage because the uterine lining can't supply adequate blood to the fetus as it grows. The deficiency commonly leads to first-trimester miscarriages.
- *Bicornuate uterus.* A woman may also have difficulty carrying her baby to full term if she has a *bicornuate,* or heart-shaped, uterus. Less common than a septate uterus,

a bicornuate uterus is a congenital anomaly that forms during the development of the female reproductive tract. The uterus fails to unify and creates two smaller cavities. (A variation is *unicornuate*, which suggests one narrow cavity, or horn.) Because the endometrial lining of a bicornuate uterus is normal, an embryo can implant and grow. But the fetus may run out of room during the second trimester, risking preterm labor and a possible premature delivery.

- *T-shaped uterus.* If your mother took a synthetic estrogen called *diethylstilbestrol* (*DES*) when she was pregnant with you, you are at risk for this uncommon congenital anomaly. Prescribed from the 1940s to the 1960s in the United States to prevent miscarriages and other abnormalities, DES not only failed to protect pregnant women, but caused birth defects and other problems in their children. Unlike a normal, rounded uterus, a T-shaped uterus is long, narrow, and underdeveloped. This formation makes it difficult for women to maintain a pregnancy beyond the first or second trimester. A T-shaped uterus also puts women at greater risk for ectopic pregnancies and cervical problems.

Cervical Factors

Cervical factors may be involved in a small percentage of female infertility cases. Located in the lower portion of the uterus, the cervix is a tight muscle opening between the vagina and the uterus that holds a fetus in place as it develops.

One potential problem is *cervical stenosis,* a condition in which the cervix becomes so tight that normal sperm passage can be difficult. Cervical stenosis often results from procedures to remove precancerous tissue. The resulting scarring can also impair cervical mucus production, which is essential for sperm transport. However, evidence is still inconclusive as to the direct effect of cervical stenosis on fertility. Cervical stenosis is not congenital, so unless you've undergone a cervical procedure, it's unlikely you'll have this condition.

A more controversial concept involves cervical mucus itself. Some medical professionals believe that the mucus can become "hostile" to sperm. They claim a woman's body can produce antibodies that "attack" sperm as if it were bacteria or some other foreign matter. Although some fertility specialists think that *antisperm antibodies* (*ASAs*) are indeed a problem in some women, others don't believe there's enough evidence to support the concept. Still, any time cervical mucus production is impaired, trouble with conception may result.

Peritoneal Factors

The *peritoneum* is the sheath of tissue that blankets your abdominal cavity, including the pelvic region. It allows adjacent organs to glide freely and thereby perform efficiently. Peritoneal problems that disrupt that interaction can cause female infertility.

Pelvic adhesions. As explained earlier, these bands of scar tissue can result from trauma—such as surgery, injury, STDs, or infections—to your ovaries, fallopian tubes, or the surrounding peritoneal tissue. The trauma causes inflammation, which promotes the growth of the adhesions. This scar tissue can pull any of your pelvic organs out of place or bind them together, either of which distorts the anatomy and can interrupt normal function.

Adhesions between your ovaries and fallopian tubes can create fertility problems. If either structure is covered with adhesions, there's no chance of an egg being released into the fallopian tube.

Endometriosis. Another disorder of the peritoneum, *endometriosis* is a condition in which the tissue that lines the uterus grows in other areas of the body—on the surfaces of the ovaries, fallopian tubes, pelvis, bladder, and/or bowel. Endometriosis affects an estimated 30 to 40 percent of female infertility patients. It often causes severe cramping, heavy bleeding, and back or ovarian pain. However, some women with severe cases of endometriosis can be pain-free; in fact, 50 percent of women have no discomfort.

Experts aren't sure what causes endometriosis, but researchers are pursuing many avenues. A common theory is that the disease develops when menstrual blood and tissue, which normally exit the body during your period, back up into the fallopian tubes. From there, the endometrial cells flow into the pelvic cavity, where they attach to the organs and surrounding tissue.

Endometriosis can affect fertility in several complicated ways. The more extensive the disease, the greater the impact on a woman's ability to get pregnant. If moderate to severe, endometriosis can distort your anatomy by causing scar tissue to develop on your reproductive organs. If your fallopian tubes are affected, it's particularly a problem—because even if you ovulate successfully, the egg has no chance of uniting with the sperm.

What's more, the disease can trigger such chronic inflammation that your body's immune or healing response is to produce pelvic adhesions and increased concentrations of infection-fighting chemicals that are toxic to your fertility. These chemicals can destroy your partner's sperm and interfere with tubal and ovarian functions; they can also harm an embryo in its early development, and they can make it difficult to carry a baby to full term. This chemical activity can also result in *endometriomas,* ovarian cysts that ooze such dark, blood-thickened material when drained that they're also referred to as *chocolate cysts.* These cysts can interfere with ovulation and, some believe, with egg development.

Unexplained Infertility

In 80 to 85 percent of cases, fertility specialists are able to identify a reason or set of reasons why a couple can't conceive. But in the other 15 to 20 percent of cases, there's no obvious cause. In those unexplained cases, testing results are often normal, or the abnormalities are so minor that they wouldn't cause infertility. Couples may have a problem with factors such as egg quality, tubal function, or sperm viability, but physicians aren't able to explain why. However, even if your infertility is unexplained, that doesn't mean you can't get pregnant.

4

Getting a Diagnosis

Perhaps, if you've not been able to conceive, you've decided to see a specialist to discover why you're not getting pregnant. Today's reproductive specialists have many ways to investigate female problems that might be hindering conception. Their diagnostic tools range from blood tests to measure hormonal levels to high-tech X-rays to examine reproductive organs. There are very few problems that can't be identified and treated. Solving the mystery begins with getting a diagnosis.

Choosing the Right Physician

Many women consult their *obstetrician-gynecologist* (*OB-GYN*) when concerns first surface, but they may need a physician trained specifically in *reproductive endocrinology and infertility*, called a *reproductive endocrinologist* (*RE*). Understanding the differences may be helpful to you in seeking out the right doctor.

Obstetricians-Gynecologists (OB-GYNs)

If you're having difficulty conceiving, talking to your obstetrician-gynecologist is a logical place to start, even if you're not sure you have a fertility problem. After four years of college and four years of medical school, OB-GYNs complete a residency for four more years, focusing entirely on women's gynecologic and reproductive health. Most OB-GYNs also become board-certified in their specialty, by amassing experience and meeting testing and other criteria.

Your OB-GYN likely will do an initial evaluation. He or she may not be prepared, however, to perform tests other than blood hormone level checks, ultrasounds, and sperm counts. At some point, you may want to work with a fertility specialist—a reproductive endocrinologist.

Reproductive Endocrinologists (REs)

Reproductive endocrinologists (REs) are usually OB-GYNs with advanced education and skills in reproductive endocrinology and infertility. In addition to completing undergraduate college and medical school, they undergo a rigorous three-year fellowship, during which they learn to manage complex problems related to female and male infertility. That includes performing high-tech procedures to uncover and treat fertility problems.

Your Doctor as Advocate

If you decide to work with a reproductive endocrinologist, choose carefully. You will want your fertility specialist to be a strong advocate in your effort to have a baby. Find a doctor who's willing to take the time to carefully explain your diagnosis and all the treatment options available to you.

Your fertility specialist should also be someone with whom you have a strong rapport. You'll want a physician who has the listening skills and compassion to make you feel comfortable. It's important that you have trust and confidence in him or her. During your first meeting with the doctor, you'll get a sense of whether you're a good match. Listen carefully to your intuition—those gut feelings are rarely wrong. If the rapport doesn't "feel right," don't hesitate to seek out another specialist.

The first step in the fertility treatment process is the initial evaluation, during which you'll provide your medical, gynecologic, obstetric, and family histories and likely have a physical examination.

Your Medical History

Your doctor will want to know your general health history. He or she should be informed of any significant medical problem or surgery. For example, if you have a chronic ailment, such as lupus, that information may be critical in deciding how to manage your care throughout a pregnancy. Also, any surgery in your abdominal or pelvic area could affect a pregnancy.

Your age won't tell your physician everything he or she needs to know about your potential for pregnancy, but it will be an indicator of the quantity and quality of your eggs.

Your Gynecologic History

Your doctor will also ask about your gynecologic history. For example, he or she will want to know if your menstrual cycle is irregular or if you've had a *tubal ligation*, endometriosis, or an ovary removed. Also, if you've undergone previous fertility evaluations, your physician may request previous test results. REs are aware that by the time many patients get to them, they may have undergone a number of expensive tests. Providing your doctor with your medical records may eliminate the need to repeat tests you've had previously.

Your Obstetric History

Your obstetric history can tell your physician much about your ability to conceive and carry a baby. Information about previous pregnancies offers important facts, as does your history with miscarriages or elective terminations. Some women are embarrassed to share that they've voluntarily interrupted, or aborted, a pregnancy. They may also be reluctant to reveal that they've had an abortion if their current partner is unaware of that. But the fact that you've been able to conceive in the past affects your doctor's current evaluation of your fertility.

Also, multiple terminations, whether abortions or miscarriages, can put you at greater risk for uterine, cervical, or tubal damage. Instruments inserted through a dilated cervix into the uterus to evacuate tissue can cause infection that leads to adhesions or other damage. By being aware of your past procedures, your doctor can recommend the most appropriate diagnostic tests for you now.

Your Family History

If your mother, grandmother, or maternal aunts had problems with conception and carrying a child, their history may be an indication of problems you may encounter. For example, if they became pregnant in their late thirties or early forties, you may be able to do the same. Your physician will want to know at what age your mother entered menopause, because that's a fairly reliable indicator of when you'll reach menopause. This information could be important if your doctor is concerned about ovarian failure or decreased ovarian reserve.

Physical Examination

Your fertility specialist may or may not perform a physical examination as part of your initial evaluation. Some physicians perform a manual exam of the pelvis, breasts, and thyroid gland. Other doctors glean what they need from your medical history. If you haven't had a gynecologic exam or Pap smear within the last year, you should have both before moving forward. Neither of these preliminaries, however, is necessary for an infertility diagnosis.

Evaluating Hormone Levels

Checking hormone levels through blood tests is one of the simplest, most noninvasive ways to begin evaluating your reproductive potential. Your hormones play a decisive role in driving your menstrual cycle and preparing your uterus for pregnancy.

Thyroid Hormones

Secreted by the pituitary gland, *thyroid-stimulating hormone* (*TSH*) stimulates your thyroid gland to produce the thyroid hormones *triiodothyronine* (*T3*) and *thyroxin* (*T4*). Both of these hormones can influence your menstrual cycle. Overproduction of T3 and T4 causes *hyperthyroidism*, more commonly known as *overactive thyroid*, while underproduction results in *hypothyroidism*, or *underactive thyroid*. A TSH test can detect both hyper- and hypothyroidism.

Prolactin

The hormone prolactin is secreted by the pituitary gland to stimulate the production of breast milk. Prolactin level is naturally elevated when a woman is pregnant or nursing. But an increase at other times can interfere with the production of estradiol and progesterone, two hormones necessary to regulate your menstrual cycle, particularly the luteal phase, when uterine changes occur. Insufficient levels of estradiol and progesterone can hinder the changes needed to support fertilization and a growing fetus. That results in difficulty with conception and/or increased risk of miscarriage.

A high prolactin level can be triggered by many factors, including hypothyroidism and tiny, slow-growing benign pituitary tumors called *microadenomas* or *prolactinomas*.

Progesterone

Some doctors order a serum progesterone test to see if a woman is ovulating normally. Produced by the ovaries in very large quantities during the luteal phase of your cycle, progesterone is responsible for a complete makeover of the uterine lining to prepare it for pregnancy. Production normally rises from preovulation to a postovulation peak. If the ovaries produce insufficient amounts, however, the uterus doesn't have the necessary ten to twelve days to prepare for sustaining a pregnancy. Measuring serum progesterone level six to seven days after midcycle can confirm whether you've ovulated and/or whether you're experiencing progesterone deficiencies that could lead to this *luteal phase defect.* (Levels greater than 3ng/ML indicate ovulation.)

Day 3 Estradiol (Estrogen)

Estradiol is the most important member of the hormone family called estrogen, which your body produces during your childbearing years. (Day 3 refers to the third day of the menstrual cycle.) As a primary sex hormone, it's critical in the manufacture of healthy, mature eggs. As such, estradiol level is often measured to gauge ovarian function and egg reserve. Your estradiol level peaks just prior to ovulation. It then drops

Female Hormones

Hormone	Function
Estradiol Estrogen	Primary sex hormone in females. Produced by the ovaries and placenta. Causes thickening of the uterine lining to accept an embryo and support a pregnancy.
FSH Follicle-stimulating hormone	Secreted by the pituitary gland. Causes an egg to mature and produce estrogen, helping to facilitate ovulation.
GnRH Gonadotropin-releasing hormone	Produced by the hypothalamus. Involved in the production of other hormones necessary for ovulation. Injectible GnRH is used to prevent spontaneous ovulation.
hCG Human chorionic gonadotropin	Produced by the placenta after fertilization. Stimulates higher levels of FSH and LH for ovulation.
LH Luteinizing hormone	Produced by the pituitary gland. Facilitates the release of a mature egg during ovulation and the production of progesterone by the corpus luteum.
Progesterone	Secreted by the ovaries, placenta, and adrenal glands. Helps release an egg each month. Causes further thickening of the uterine lining to support a growing embryo during pregnancy. Helps maintain sufficient blood flow to the fetus.
Prolactin	Secreted by the pituitary gland. Causes milk production in the breasts and transport to the ducts.
TSH Thyroid-stimulating hormone	Secreted by the pituitary gland. Tells the thyroid to produce the thyroid hormones T3 (triiodothyronine) and T4 (thyroxin), both of which influence the menstrual cycle.

dramatically, signaling release of an egg. As with progesterone, the level of estradiol rises in anticipation of fertilization, but falls abruptly if pregnancy doesn't occur within ten to twelve days.

Day 3 Follical-Stimulating Hormone (FSH)

Follicle-stimulating hormone (FSH) is also necessary for producing healthy eggs. Yet a higher-than-normal FSH level can signal premature ovarian failure (POF) or age-related diminished ovarian reserve, which could affect reproductive function. Since FSH and luteinizing hormone (LH) work together in triggering egg production, doctors often test these hormone levels at the same time.

Day 3 Luteinizing Hormone (LH)

Released by the pituitary gland, luteinizing hormone (LH) stimulates ovulation by surging. Once the egg has been released, LH then activates the transformation of the empty, collapsed follicle into a new structure called the corpus luteum. This structure secretes progesterone and, to a lesser extent, estradiol during the second half of a woman's cycle. A higher-than-normal level of LH early in the cycle can indicate menstrual disorders. In a fertility evaluation, an LH test is often done along with other hormone tests, even though the results are not always as useful.

Endometrial Biopsy

An *endometrial biopsy* is sometimes helpful in determining whether the lining of your uterus (the endometrium) is developing during your ovulatory cycle and preparing to sustain a pregnancy. The test involves removing a small sample of endometrial tissue from the uterus after ovulation—one to three days before your period begins—and then examining it under a microscope to see if the cells are undergoing the proper luteal phase changes.

Performed in your doctor's office, the procedure to remove the tissue is similar to that used for a Pap smear. In this case, however, the physician gently slips a strawlike sheath through the cervix into the uterus to suction a sample of the lining tissue.

From start to finish, the procedure should take only a few minutes, with the actual tissue removal requiring less than sixty seconds. Relatively painless, the procedure will not increase your risk of miscarriage if you're already pregnant.

Doctors always perform an endometrial biopsy if they suspect a luteal phase defect. However, many physicians believe the test is far more useful in investigating the cause of recurrent miscarriages than in evaluating fertility.

Evaluating the Reproductive Organs

Your doctor also needs to know if your reproductive organs are working normally and are ready for conception, pregnancy, and childbirth. Physicians have several ways to examine the ovaries, fallopian tubes, uterus, and cervix.

Pelvic and Transvaginal Ultrasound

Used widely in obstetrics and gynecology, ultrasound offers a quick view of your abdominal and pelvic cavities. A painless procedure, ultrasound works by sending high-frequency sound waves into your body through a device called a *transducer*, which is rotated over your abdomen or inserted into your vagina. As the sound waves bounce off soft-tissue structures, they produce echoes, which are then detected, analyzed, and converted by a computer into images on a screen.

Although pelvic and transvaginal ultrasounds are frequently used to monitor pregnancies, they're a useful, noninvasive tool in diagnosing infertility, too. Your doctor may order an ultrasound to examine your uterus and ovaries or to track follicular growth after you've taken fertility drugs.

Saline-Infusion Sonohysterography (SIS)

Saline-infusion sonohysterography (*SIS*) allows your doctor to examine the uterine cavity and its lining for tiny polyps, fibroids, adhesions, and other abnormalities. (This test is also known as a *sonohysterogram,* or *SHG.*)

Performed in your doctor's office using ultrasound imaging, the test involves opening the vagina with a speculum and threading a small catheter through the cervix and into the uterus. As the speculum is removed, a vaginal ultrasound probe replaces it. Sterile saline, or saltwater, solution is then slowly infused into the uterus through the catheter. The solution slowly and gently expands the space, allowing your physician to see any defects or growths such as polyps and fibroids. Most women tolerate SIS very well; however, you may feel cramping as the catheter is inserted and your uterus fills with liquid.

Hysterosalpingography (HSG)

Another test used to examine the uterine cavity as well as the fallopian tubes is *hysterosalpingography* (*HSG*). One of the most useful nonsurgical tools for diagnosing infertility, HSG combines sophisticated X-ray technology with a dye solution, so that your physician is able to view polyps and fibroids in your uterus and see whether your fallopian tubes are structurally normal.

HSG is usually performed between days seven and eleven of your cycle, after you've stopped menstruating and before you've ovulated. Your doctor must work within that window, or risk either flushing an egg out of the fallopian tube or irradiating a developing embryo. To perform this procedure, he or she inserts a narrow catheter through the cervix into the uterus. A dye solution is then injected slowly into the uterus through the catheter. X-rays are taken to mark the dye's progression as it fills the uterus and flows through the fallopian tubes. Your doctor can easily see the outline of your tubes and determine whether the dye exits into your pelvis. If it does not, you likely have a tubal obstruction.

How well you tolerate HSG depends largely on whether or not your tubes are blocked. If your doctor needs to inject the dye more forcefully, you'll probably feel increased cramping. Fortunately, taking ibuprofen or a similar painkiller before and after the procedure usually alleviates discomfort. Antibiotics are sometimes prescribed for several days in advance of the test to reduce the risk of infection, which is less than 2 percent.

Hysteroscopy

A *hysteroscopy* is performed by threading a tiny, fiber-optically-lit telescope through the cervix into the uterus. The uterus is then expanded with saline solution or carbon dioxide gas so that the doctor can see the entire cavity clearly. Some physicians use diagnostic hysteroscopy to detect smaller polyps and fibroids that aren't necessarily evident with HSG. The procedure is also useful in treating abnormalities—such as removing polyps, adhesions, or fibroids without damaging healthy tissue.

Both diagnostic and operative hysteroscopies are usually performed in an outpatient surgical center, but they may be done in an office setting. Depending on the extent of the problem, you'll be given a local anesthetic, mild sedation, or even general anesthesia. Most women tolerate the procedure well.

Laparoscopy

Laparoscopy offers another way of examining and treating your ovaries, uterus, and fallopian tubes. Laparoscopy uses a long, thin, fiber-optically-lit tube, threaded through a small incision in your navel, to identify certain fertility problems and even correct them at the same time they're diagnosed. As part of the procedure, carbon dioxide gas is pumped into the abdominal cavity to expand the space, providing a better view for the doctor.

Because laparoscopy is performed under general anesthesia, it's usually used only if a problem can't be diagnosed with other tests or needs to be corrected with the procedure. By manipulating other tools through one or two small incisions, your doctor can burn or cut away adhesions, fibroids, ovarian cysts, or endometriosis lesions. (One incision is made in the navel, and one is made just above the pubic bone.) Although recovery is usually relatively quick, some women experience abdominal bloating and tenderness for a day or so.

Other Blood Tests

Your fertility specialist can learn many things from blood tests besides how your hormones are fluctuating and whether you're ovulating. Other blood tests check for Chlamydia infection, German measles, chicken pox, and hepatitis, as well as disorders such as *antiphospholipid antibodies (APAs), lupus anticoagulants, gene mutations,* and antisperm antibodies (ASAs). Although some of the information obtained from these tests may not be relevant in terms of your ability to conceive, it can be very relevant in terms of your ability to carry a baby to full term.

Chlamydia Infection

Your doctor may order a blood test for Chlamydia infection if he or she suspects tubal damage related to the infection. (Your tubes may appear open on an X-ray, but still be unable to move or pick up an egg because of infection-related adhesions.) A standard blood test detects only a current, active Chlamydia infection, so your physician may want a blood antibody test. An antibody test can reveal signs of a past infection, which may have caused adhesions and/or microscopic injury.

By knowing that you were exposed to Chlamydia infection at some point, your doctor may test your fallopian tubes. With every Chlamydia exposure, there's a 25 percent chance of tubal problems as well as an increased risk for a tubal (ectopic) pregnancy. If you're already pregnant, you'll be monitored routinely with ultrasound to ensure the embryo remains in the uterus.

German Measles and Chicken Pox

You may also have antibody blood tests to check your immunity to German measles (rubella) and chicken pox (varicella). You may have lost your immunity to these diseases as you've grown older. Contracting either of them during your first trimester of pregnancy can cause birth defects and have other devastating effects on the fetus.

Hepatitis B and C

Your doctor may also order blood tests to determine whether either of these viruses is active in your body. Both viruses can cause chronic and sometimes life-threatening inflammation of the liver. Your body should be able to fight either virus with antibodies, but a baby's immune system can't handle the assault.

Since a mild case of hepatitis B, in particular, may be mistaken for the flu, it can go undetected. This can be particularly dangerous if missed during pregnancy, because there's a 5 to 12 percent risk that you'll pass the disease along to your baby. By knowing whether the hepatitis B virus is active in your body, your doctor can make sure that your baby is vaccinated at birth. Since there's no hepatitis C vaccination, you need to make sure you don't have an active case if you're trying to conceive.

Antiphospholipid Antibodies (APAs)

Phospholipids are fatty materials found in the walls of all blood vessels. But some women, especially those having problems conceiving, produce antiphospholipid antibodies (APAs). These special proteins can attack and damage blood vessel walls, causing micro-clots during healing. In major blood vessels, these small clots are of no consequence. But in the tiny vessels of a developing fetus, they can be large enough to block the flow of blood. This can lead to pregnancy loss between ovulation and your period—or worse, a miscarriage between the sixth and eighth weeks, when there's an increased demand from the fetus for nutrients from the blood.

Routine testing for antiphospholipid antibodies is controversial. The argument against it is that fertile women can test positive but have no problems conceiving or carrying a baby to full term. Many fertility specialists, therefore, don't offer this testing unless a woman has a history of two or more miscarriages. Other doctors, however, believe that performing the test initially may prevent the emotional and physical trauma of multiple miscarriages for some women. The test is recommended if you have a history of major *deep* or *superficial venous thrombosis* (blood clotting in the veins), even if you have never miscarried.

Lupus Anticoagulants

If your physician chooses to test for antiphospholipid antibodies, he or she may also check for lupus anticoagulants. These antibodies can cause small blood clots to form in the placenta, preventing the fetus from getting proper nutrition. Although the term *lupus* suggests that these anticoagulants have something to do with the chronic inflammatory immune disorder also known as *lupus,* the two are not related. It's also a bit of a misnomer to call these antibodies *anticoagulants,* since they don't prevent blood from clotting. (They simply look like anticoagulants in the lab.) Instead, they behave like antiphospholipid antibodies, which is really what they are. Unless your doctor diagnoses lupus anticoagulants through a blood test and treats the disorder with medication, you might experience repeated miscarriages or premature delivery.

Factor V Leiden

An inherited disorder, the *factor V Leiden* gene mutation can cause abnormal blood clotting, which in turn can cause a variety of problems during pregnancy, most notably miscarriage. Normally, the body produces a clotting protein, called *factor V,* that helps with healing. The body also manufactures anticlotting enzymes to keep the clotting in check. In individuals with the factor V Leiden gene mutation, factor V's response to the anticlotting enzymes is slower, which can result in excess clotting.

If blood clots occur, your doctor will treat you with *warfarin (Coumadin),* a blood thinner, if you aren't pregnant. If you are trying to conceive, the doctor will likely prescribe a quick-acting, injectable blood thinner called *heparin.* You'll be monitored closely once you're pregnant, to see that clotting times are within the normal range.

Methylenetetrahydrofolate Reductase (MTHFR) Deficiency

Another gene mutation, *methylenetetrahydrofolate reductase (MTHFR) deficiency* can create problems during pregnancy by raising the level of the amino acid homocysteine. An elevated level of homocysteine is associated with *preeclampsia,* a form of high blood pressure that may develop during pregnancy. The enzyme deficiency can lead to miscarriages and possible spinal cord defects. By lowering your homocysteine level with B vitamins, folic acid, and baby aspirin, however, you can lower your risk of miscarriage.

Antisperm Antibodies (ASAs)

Testing for antisperm antibodies (ASAs) is based on the premise that conception can't occur if a woman's cervical mucus is "hostile" to her partner's sperm. That is, her body actually has an allergic or immune reaction to sperm and produces "indirect" antisperm antibodies—special proteins that can immobilize sperm and prevent them from fertilizing an egg. If your doctor suspects that you have a mucus-sperm interaction problem or can't explain your infertility, he or she may order an antisperm antibody test.

Some doctors question the validity of the concept that a woman's cervical mucus can even be hostile to sperm. Still others question the usefulness of ASA testing. These critics suggest that since fewer than 5 percent of all females have an allergic reaction to semen, it's unlikely that the antibodies cause infertility. They also point out that a doctor can bypass antibodies that might be lurking in the cervical mucus by creating embryos in the lab and then implanting them directly in the uterus.

If you're about to undergo *intrauterine insemination (IUI),* a procedure in which sperm is deposited in the uterus, however, your doctor may suggest the test. If the ASA theory holds true, then indirect ASAs can exist anywhere in the reproductive tract and thus can prevent conception even if your partner's sperm is placed into the uterus through IUI. In other words, you may be bypassing the cervical mucus but still have a problem.

Some doctors find low-dose prednisone to be effective in lowering the percentage of antibodies working against the sperm, thus allowing for conception naturally or through IUI. But whether the benefits outweigh the risks is a topic of controversy. In any case, ASA testing may be used sooner rather than later, to (hopefully) eliminate ASAs as an underlying problem.

Postcoital Testing (PCT)

Commonly used in the past, *postcoital testing (PCT)* plays a smaller role in diagnosing female infertility today. Some doctors still use it to see if a woman's cervical mucus is viable and if her partner's sperm is functioning within the mucus. Your cervical mucus changes throughout your cycle, from thick and milky to thin and clear at ovulation (when it needs to facilitate sperm transport). The mucus may not be viable or hospitable to sperm, however, if your cervix is damaged by previous procedures or even affected by the anti-estrogen effects of oral fertility drugs.

Postcoital testing is performed soon after intercourse, prior to ovulation. Although there are various ways to time the test, the most accurate method is to monitor a woman's follicles with ultrasound until they reach a mature size—usually, 18 millimeters. Within two to twelve hours of intercourse, the doctor obtains a sample of the woman's cervical mucus by threading a catheter into her cervix. The sperm within the mucus is evaluated microscopically for consistency, elasticity, and motility, or forward movement.

The criticisms of postcoital testing are that there's little standardization in how it's performed, read, or interpreted, and no agreement on what constitutes a good-versus-bad result.

At-Home Tests

Charts for recording *basal body temperature (BBT)* and over-the-counter *ovulation-predictor kits* (OPKs) have become standard natural planning tools for many women trying to get pregnant.

The BBT test requires you to record your basal, or "at rest," temperature before getting out of bed every morning during an entire menstrual cycle. The test is supposed to pinpoint a good time to conceive, because your body temperature drops right before ovulation and rises distinctively once an egg is released.

OPKs predict the next time you will ovulate by measuring your LH level (which surges before ovulation). To measure LH, you dip a test strip into an early-morning urine sample; the strip either turns a color or displays a plus sign if an LH surge is detected. If that occurs, you should ovulate within the next twenty-four to forty hours—the window of opportunity for conception.

Some doctors use BBT charts and OPKs as quick and inexpensive checks for ovulation. But the accuracy of these tests is totally dependent on whether they're used correctly. Also, compared to other, verifiable tests, BBT and OPKs are relatively unreliable.

5

Treatment with Fertility Drugs

ertility drugs are the first line of treatment for many women who wish to become pregnant. This array of potent medications, both oral and injectable, can regulate a woman's menstrual cycle, stimulate ovulation, and improve egg quality. These drugs are used in 80 to 85 percent of female infertility cases.

Clomiphene Citrate

The most commonly prescribed drug for women with an impaired ovulatory cycle is *clomiphene citrate*. Sold in the United States under the trade name *Clomid* or *Serophene*, it's an inexpensive oral medication used to stimulate a normal cycle in women with irregular or absent periods. The drug mimics hormones, so that the resulting cycle behaves very much like a natural cycle in how long it takes to "recruit" and develop a single follicle for ovulation. As such, clomiphene citrate is considered the mildest of fertility medications, even though it must be used judiciously and under close monitoring. It's typically prescribed as a 50-milligram tablet taken once daily for five days, starting between cycle days three and five.

If you're not having periods, your doctor may order either an oral progestin (such as *Provera*) or an injectable natural progesterone to induce bleeding first. If you don't menstruate after taking the drug, you're not a candidate for clomiphene citrate; if given the medication, you probably won't respond.

Women on clomiphene citrate are usually monitored with ultrasound to track follicle growth and/or with blood tests to measure progesterone levels. If ovulation doesn't occur after the first month, the dosage can be increased in 50 milligram increments over subsequent cycles. Because clomiphene citrate blocks estradiol receptors in the brain, its use can reduce the cervical mucus necessary for sperm to swim to the uterus, which will impede conception. Use of this drug also can decrease uterine lining thickness, interfering with implantation of the fertilized egg. Clomiphene citrate should be used only in fertility treatment; it should not be given to women who are ovulating normally and simply want to boost their chances of getting pregnant.

Although clomiphene citrate induces ovulation in 80 percent of women with ovulatory dysfunction and no other fertility issues, only 50 to 60 percent conceive. Of those who get pregnant, 85 percent do so within three cycles; 95 percent do so within six cycles. About 8 percent of women become pregnant with multiples, usually twins.

Although clomiphene citrate is generally well tolerated, side effects can include menopausal-like symptoms, which usually disappear after treatment ends. In those rare cases when headaches or visual problems occur, the drug must be discontinued and, usually, never used again.

Injectable Gonadotropins

Another mainstay in fertility treatment, *injectable gonadotropins*, are considerably more powerful than clomiphene citrate in stimulating the ovaries. Using these high-powered injections creates *controlled ovarian hyperstimulation.* That is, the drugs stimulate the ovaries to produce more quality eggs in a shorter period of time. Normally, a woman's body selects one egg follicle each month and nurtures it until she ovulates. However, with injectable gonadotropins, a woman's ovulatory system is *hyperstimulated* to dramatically increase her egg production and per-cycle probability of conception.

In virtually all cases, women must give themselves the injections (or have their partners give them) because they must be given once or twice a day, with one always given at night. Your doctor's staff will instruct you on how to give yourself the injections. Most women or their partners quickly become adept at giving themselves the shots.

Most often, the injectable medications are given subcutaneously, or under the skin. Subcutaneous shots can be given anywhere on the body, but are most commonly given in the abdomen or the front of the thigh. Because a thin needle is used, most women do not find these shots painful.

A few of the medications must be injected intramuscularly, or into the muscle, usually in the hip or the front of the thigh. These shots must be given with a larger needle and may be more painful than subcutaneous injections.

Human menopausal gonadotropin (hMG). This commonly used injectable gonadotropin contains equal parts of follicle-stimulating hormone (FSH) and luteinizing hormone (LH), the pituitary hormones that stimulate the ovaries to produce mature eggs. Many doctors commonly use injectable hMG because it's a simple regimen that consistently produces good results. It not only replicates the action of FSH, but also of LH—which, in a natural cycle, surges to set ovulation in motion. Brand names include *Pergonal, Menopur,* and *Repronex.*

Injectable hMG is used in conjunction with timed intercourse, intrauterine insemination (IUI), and in vitro fertilization (IVF). Although hMG regimens vary, the patient usually administers an injection once or twice daily over six to twelve days. Patients are monitored closely during treatment.

Side effects of hMG may include minor breast and abdominal tenderness. There is also a risk of conceiving multiples. Approximately 15 to 20 percent of women using hMG will have multiple births, usually twins.

However, the greatest concern with hMG is the risk of excessive stimulation called *ovarian hyperstimulation syndrome (OHSS)*, which occurs in approximately 1 percent of patients taking hMG. However, with judicious ultrasound monitoring, multiples and OHSS are not likely to be problems.

Commonly Used Fertility Drugs

Generic Names	Brand Names	Delivery Method
Clomiphene citrate	Clomid, Serophene	Pill
HMG		
Follicle-stimulating hormone–luteinizing hormone	Menopur, Repronex Pergonal	Injection(subcutaneous) Injection(intramuscular)
FSH		
Follicle-stimulating hormone	Follistim, Gonal-F, Bravelle	Injection (subcutaneous)
HCG		
Chorionic gonadotropin	Novarel, Pregnyl Ovidrel	Injection (intramuscular) Injection (subcutaneous)
GnRH Agonists		
Leuprolide acetate	Lupron	Injection (subcutaneous)
GnRH Antagonists		
Ganirelex acetate	Antagon	Injection (subcutaneous)
Cetrorelix acetate	Cetrotide	Injection (subcutaneous)
Progesterone		
Injectable		Injection (intramuscular)
Vaginal gel	Crinone	Applied intravaginally
Vaginal tablet	Endometrin	Inserted manually
Medication	Prometrium	Pill

Follicle-stimulating hormone (FSH). This drug is often prescribed for women who do not respond to clomiphene therapy. These injections contain FSH and very little LH. FSH drugs such as *Follistim, Gonal-F,* and *Bravelle* are injected subcutaneously. These medications are well tolerated and produce excellent results.

Human chorionic gonadotropin (hCG). These injections help fertility specialists precisely control when a woman's ovaries release a mature egg for fertilization. Nearly identical in chemical structure and function to natural LH, hCG replicates the body's natural LH surge. When sufficient mature follicles are detected on an ultrasound, the doctor injects hCG to trigger, or induce, ovulation. As with natural LH, hCG ensures that an egg completes the final *meiotic* divisions necessary to mature. It also helps the follicle remodel itself into the corpus luteum and manufacture progesterone.

Injectable hCG is manufactured under the trade names *Novarel* and *Pregnyl* (injected intramuscularly), *Ovidrel* (injected subcutaneously), and many others.

In addition to the lead-up to in vitro fertilization, hCG is used prior to timed intercourse and intrauterine insemination. In any case, ovulation occurs close to eight to forty hours after an hCG trigger shot. The precise time of ovulation is monitored with both ultrasound and blood estradiol tests. Human chorionic gonadotropin is tolerated well and produces excellent results.

Potential Complication of Ovarian Hyperstimulation

An uncommon yet potentially serious complication, ovarian hyperstimulation syndrome (OHSS), occurs if ovarian hyperstimulation is excessive. Because of the risk, women using injectable gonadotropins must be monitored even more closely than those taking clomiphene citrate.

OHSS can vary from mild to severe or critical. Often, the first signs of the syndrome are significantly enlarged and painful ovaries, which may rupture and bleed. In more advanced cases, women experience shifting, or leaking, of fluids from the ovarian blood vessels into the abdomen. In addition to triggering significant weight gain within days, this fluid shift can result in a range of symptoms from nausea to shortness of breath. It can also upset the normal blood chemistry and balance of the body, putting a woman at risk for potentially life-threatening problems such as unstable blood pressure, blood clots, and kidney failure.

Fortunately, less than 1 percent of women who experience OHSS have symptoms severe enough to be hospitalized. Most women can be treated successfully with fluid and electrolyte replacements at home. With appropriate treatment, this disorder usually corrects itself within two weeks, and pregnancy outcomes are usually very good.

Other Fertility Drugs

Gonadotropin-Releasing Hormone (GnRH) Agonists

The *gonadotropin-releasing hormone (GnRH) agonists* mimic natural GnRH in controlling a woman's ovulatory cycle so that it responds appropriately for IVF. Natural GnRH switches on a woman's cycle by stimulating the pituitary gland to secrete FSH and LH. These hormones, in turn, cause the ovaries to recruit follicles, develop eggs, and release eggs. Although GnRH agonists, such as *leuprolide acetate* (*Lupron*), can play several roles in fertility treatment, the most common is to control a woman's cycle so that she doesn't prematurely or spontaneously release eggs just prior to IVF. By preventing her natural LH surge, GnRH agonists prevent ovulation, which allows the eggs to be retrieved for an IVF cycle.

GnRH agonists are injected subcutaneously in a controlled regimen based on a woman's age and reproductive history as well as her physician's preferences.

Gonadotropin-Releasing Hormone (GnRH) Antagonists

Newer and faster-acting than GnRH agonists, *gonado-tropin-releasing hormone (GnRH) antagonists* also prevent a spontaneous LH surge during the stimulation leading up to egg retrieval for IVF. Unlike GnRH agonists, however, GnRH antagonists prohibit a woman from making or releasing FSH and LH altogether.

Given subcutaneously, GnRH antagonists, such as *ganirelex acetate* (*Antagon*) and *cetrorelix acetate* (*Cetrotide*), prevent spontaneous ovulation with far less medication and without exhausting the pituitary. Quick and direct, these drugs can shut down the pituitary with one injection, which means patients don't have to take injections for weeks as they do with GnRH agonists. Instead, the pituitary operates normally until that very moment when it must produce an LH surge. Despite these advantages, some fertility specialists don't prescribe GnRH antagonists, because unlike GnRH agonists, they can't be used for non-IVF issues, such as treating endometriosis. But for IVF purposes, they do produce comparable results.

Supplemental Progesterone

Women often receive supplemental progesterone after fertility treatment to enhance their chances that an embryo will implant and the fetus will survive to full term. Produced in large quantities during the luteal phase of a normal cycle, progesterone is needed to prepare the uterus for pregnancy. But some women don't make enough of the hormone to trigger the changes to the uterine lining (endometrium) that are necessary to support the fetus. Having this luteal phase defect doesn't necessarily mean that you're likely to miscarry; it simply means that you fall into a group more likely to have problems—which often can be prevented with supplemental progesterone.

The most likely candidates for supplemental progesterone are women with a history of two or three miscarriages or with luteal phases consistently lasting less than eleven days. Progesterone is also given almost universally with in vitro fertilization.

Supplemental progesterone can be administered in several forms, including intramuscular injections, vaginal suppositories, topic gels, tablets, or capsules. Progesterone supplements are usually tolerated well by most women.

6

Fertility Treatment Procedures

In 1978, Louise Brown of Great Britain became the first so-called test-tube baby. Her birth ushered in a new era in fertility treatment: in vitro fertilization, or IVF. Since then, millions of couples have had babies thanks to IVF, the centerpiece of a group of fertility treatments known as *assisted reproductive technologies* (*ARTs*).

In this chapter, we'll discuss the various ART treatments available today along with other treatments, including intrauterine insemination cryopreservation, which involves the freezing of sperm, eggs, and embryos.

Intrauterine Insemination (IUI)

Intrauterine insemination, or IUI, involves impregnating a woman by injecting her partner's sperm directly into her uterus. The procedure offers couples, particularly those facing male or cervical factor infertility, an effective treatment option. IUI is often recommended when:

- a male partner has a decrease in sperm count or quality or has difficulty with erection or ejaculation
- a woman lacks cervical mucus because of damage to the cervix, or the interaction between her mucus and sperm is poor
- a couple wants an aggressive alternative to timed intercourse but doesn't need IVF
- infertility is unexplained

IUI can be performed in conjunction with a woman's natural cycle, but it's usually done when she's undergone ovulation induction, to give her partner's sperm a better chance of impregnating an egg. Although oral drugs can be used, many fertility specialists prefer low-dose hMG or FSH injections to stimulate egg production. Besides yielding two to five eggs, these drugs may result in better-quality eggs and a better hormonal environment for pregnancy. Together, these factors should produce quicker, more successful results.

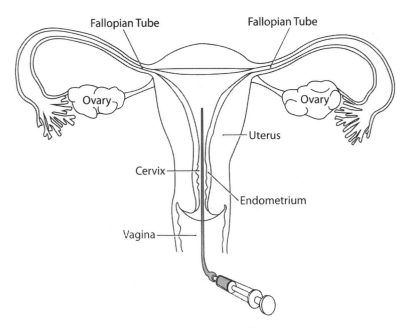

For intrauterine insemination, sperm is injected into the uterus.

Because synchronizing your partner's sperm collection with your cycle is key in IUI, your fertility specialist will monitor the development of your follicles with transvaginal ultrasound every two or three days. When the lead follicles are mature, he or she will trigger ovulation, usually with injectable hCG. Doctors like this drug because of its predictability in stimulating the release of a mature egg within thirty-eight hours of the injection. When ovulation is imminent, your partner will give a semen sample, which is then washed. The washing does the same job as the cervical mucus—it separates the strongest sperm from the weakest. The sperm is then placed in the uterine cavity via a special catheter.

An IUI procedure is performed in a doctor's office. Other than mild cramping, side effects are uncommon; most women find IUI to be a relatively quick and pain-free procedure. Because there is a 15 to 20 percent risk of multiples (usually twins), doctors track the number of follicles with ultrasound. If they see too many, they cancel the treatment cycle.

Success rates with IUI vary widely, depending on the number of normal motile sperm available, the type of drugs used for ovarian stimulation, and any female factors involved. Because the probability for success varies, your doctor will discuss whether IUI is recommended for you. Although it takes an average of three or four attempts to succeed with IUI, fertility specialists usually recommend no more than six tries, since success isn't likely after that point. But for couples who are likely to be successful in two or three attempts, this procedure offers a less costly and less stressful option than procedures involving advanced reproductive technology.

If you're planning to undergo IUI or any high-tech fertility treatment, your doctor will likely recommend that both you and your partner be tested for communicable diseases, including syphilis, human immunodeficiency virus (HIV), hepatitis B and C, mycoplasma, and Chlamydia infection. The Food and Drug Administration (FDA) requires this testing of all egg and sperm donors, and the testing is recommended even if couples are using their own eggs and sperm.

In Vitro Fertilization (IVF)

In vitro fertilization (IVF) is a procedure in which a woman's eggs are removed from her ovaries, fertilized in a laboratory, and then transferred back into her body. With an overall success rate of about 50 percent or more (depending on

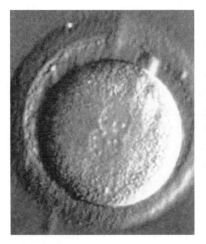 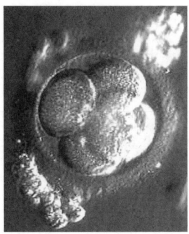

The left photo shows a fertilized egg 24 hours after IVF. The photo on the right shows a four-cell embryo two days later.

a doctor's skill, a woman's age, and other factors), IVF offers a promising path to pregnancy.

Two decades ago, only a handful of fertility clinics performed IVF and related procedures, but today, more than four hundred centers in the United States alone offer at least IVF to help couples get pregnant. Although refined over the past years, the procedure still involves the same basic steps: A woman's ovaries are hyperstimulated with fertility drugs. Her eggs are removed through the vagina, under the guidance of ultrasound. They're evaluated, fertilized with sperm, and transferred into her uterus. The remaining embryos are frozen for future use.

Inducing Follicle Development and Egg Maturation

The first step in IVF is to maximize the number of eggs you produce with injectable fertility medications. Injectable gonadotropins are preferred to oral medications because of their potency in producing many eggs. The older you are, the higher the dosages and the longer the regimens you may need to get maximum results.

Many doctors will monitor a woman's progress by using a blood estradiol test or LH test to predict whether the eggs are good enough to trigger ovulation or to ensure that she hasn't spontaneously ovulated after taking the medication. Doctors also monitor the follicles with ultrasound. Once the follicles reach a mature size of approximately 18 millimeters, a woman receives an injection of human chorionic gonadotropin (hCG). By replacing her natural surge of luteinizing hormone (LH), the injection triggers the final stage of egg maturation. Within the next thirty-six hours, the eggs should be ready for removal. Typically, doctors hope to retrieve five to fifteen eggs.

Retrieving Eggs

Retrieving eggs for IVF is usually accomplished during an outpatient surgical procedure. Many women receive light sedation for this procedure. To retrieve the eggs, the doctor inserts an ultrasound-guided needle through the back of the vaginal wall into the ovary. Once a follicle is punctured, the egg and surrounding fluid are gently sucked into an accompanying tube. The process is repeated until both ovaries are emptied.

When performed by an experienced fertility specialist, the procedure usually takes less than thirty minutes—often as few as five to ten minutes. It might take longer, however, if there are unusually large numbers of eggs or significant anatomic abnormalities. The eggs are preserved at body temperature and transferred to the lab.

Examining Eggs

Next, an embryologist (a scientist who specializes in embryo development) will examine and prepare the eggs. Using a narrow tube called a pipette, the embryologist gently sucks each egg from its follicular fluid and places it in a small, shallow dish called a petri dish, which is warmed to body temperature. Because eggs are sometimes immature at retrieval, they're confined at first to an incubator. After five or six hours, the embryologist checks their development. Mature eggs are easy to identify by the presence of a polar body, a small round structure in the wall of the egg, only produced if the egg is mature. The

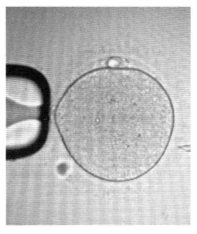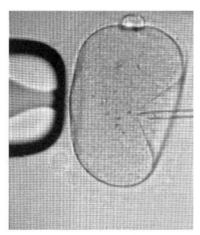

Intracytoplasmic sperm injection (ICSI) involves the injection of a single sperm into a single egg. In the left photo, a pipette (on the left) holds the egg. Photo on the right shows a needle, ready to deposit the sperm.

presence of this polar body signals that the egg is mature and ready to be fertilized.

Fertilizing Eggs

Fertilizing eggs with IVF is straightforward. Within hours of the egg retrieval, a man's sperm is collected fresh or is thawed if it has been frozen. After preparation, it's mixed with the eggs in a petri dish and incubated overnight.

Although IVF typically involves mixing thousands of sperm with the eggs in hopes of conception, it can be more focused with *intracytoplasmic sperm injection (ICSI)*. This procedure involves injecting a single sperm into a single egg. ICSI has greatly increased IVF fertilization rates. It's used in about 60 percent of all ART cycles. Many IVF clinics do it routinely to improve fertilization rates and increase the number of embryos.

The first signs of fertilization are the production of two separate round bodies, or *pronuclei,* in the center of every egg. Each pronucleus contains twenty-three chromosomes, the DNA blueprint contributed by each parent. Before the end of the first day, the pronuclei merge into one nucleus containing all forty-six chromosomes necessary for a new embryo. They grow from a single cell to eight cells by day three, reaching the final *blastocyst* (early embyro) stage by day five, when the placenta and fetal tissues separate. The embryos are monitored until transfer to the uterus, to ensure that they exhibit no developmental abnormalities. The embryologist picks the best embryos for implantation by scoring them according to their number of cells, the presence of irregularities, and their symmetry.

Transferring Embryos

Embryo transfer is a relatively quick in-office procedure. It does not require anesthesia, but some women request a mild sedative. Usually guided by ultrasound, the doctor gently threads a sterile thin plastic catheter into the uterus. Attached to it is a syringe carrying one or more embryos. Once the tip of the catheter reaches the proper part of the uterine cavity, the doctor releases the contents of the syringe. The actual IVF transfer usually takes less than thirty seconds.

Your physician will prescribe medication after the procedure. Some doctors prefer to prescribe progesterone, to assist with endometrial development and help prevent miscarriage. But others use different drugs that they believe will improve implantation and pregnancy rates: antibiotics to protect against infection; low-dose prednisone or other steroids to protect the embryo from any inflammation caused by inserting a catheter into the uterus; and baby aspirin to prevent possible micro-clotting.

Improving Success Rates

In refining their IVF methods, fertility specialists and embryologists have devised various laboratory techniques to improve success rates. Before an embryo even leaves the petri dish, for example, they can change its course by either delaying the transfer or assisting the implantation with a microscopic technique.

Blastocyst Transfer

Many women have better success with implantation if their embryos reach the final development phase, the blastocyst stage, before being transferred to the uterus. Blastocyst transfer is possible today because embryos are immersed from days three to five in a special growth medium that mimics uterine fluid, facilitating development. The thinking is that only the best embryos will reach blastocyst stage during this waiting period. That means fewer will be transferred, which diminishes the risk of multiple gestations while improving pregnancy rates. Blastocyst transfer is reserved for women who meet certain criteria, such as being under age forty with no previous failed IVF attempts but a good number of day three embryos.

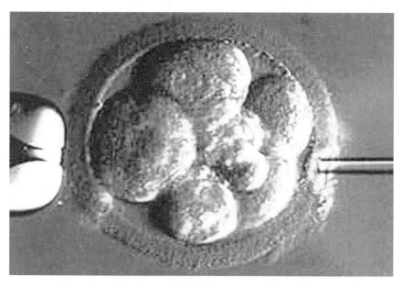

Assisted hatching helps an embryo break through the embryo wall. The pipette on the left holds the embryo while a needle on the right deposits a mild acid, which weakens the wall.

Assisted Hatching

Assisted hatching is a microscopic procedure used to help an embryo break out of its eggshell-like outer wall so that it can implant in the uterine wall. Assisted hatching is performed when the outer wall grows abnormally thick, which often occurs as a woman ages or as a result of embryo freezing. By injecting a mild, harmless acid into the shell or piercing the shell with a laser, an embryologist creates a microscopic hole that cracks open easily on implantation. That allows the embryo to "hatch" out and attach to the uterine lining.

Assisted hatching is somewhat controversial, because doctors don't universally agree on when it should be used. Although it may be helpful in selected cases, it may be detrimental in others. When doctors do recommend it, it's usually for women who are over age thirty-eight and therefore at greater risk for a hardened shell, who have experienced repeated IVF failures, who have elevated follicle-stimulating hormone (FSH) levels, or who are using frozen embryos.

Since there's a possibility of injury to the embryo, complications to the fetus, or the potential of identical twins, only a properly trained embryologist should perform assisted hatching. Also, pregnancy rates vary with each lab, so you need to ask

Fertility Treatment Procedures

ART	**assisted reproductive technologies**—procedure in which eggs are removed from a woman's body and then treated to help with conception; includes IVF, GIFT, and ZIFT
IUI	**intrauterine insemination**—washed sperm is threaded through the cervix and into the uterus, where it's delivered to fertilize eggs
IVF	**in vitro fertilization**—primary procedure for fertilizing eggs in the laboratory and then implanting the resulting embryos in the uterus
ICSI	**intracytoplasmic sperm injection**—injection of a single sperm directly into the center of an egg
GIFT	**gamete intrafallopian tube transfer**—placement of both sperm and egg directly into a woman's fallopian tubes for conception
ZIFT	**zygote intrafallopian tube transfer**—fertilization of eggs in the laboratory, followed by implantation in the fallopian tubes

about the success and complication rates if your fertility specialist suggests this procedure.

Preventing Multiples

Your doctor will recommend the number of embryos to transfer based on his or her professional experience. He or she will also follow guidelines based on your age and reproductive history. A woman's chances of having a baby improve, up to a point, as more embryos are transferred into the uterus. But the goal is to maximize the chances of pregnancy without producing high-order multiple pregnancies. This is important, because with each additional fetus, there's a greater chance of premature delivery and lifelong health problems for the baby, such as cerebral palsy, which is associated with being underdeveloped at birth. Moreover, preeclampsia (pregnancy-induced high blood pressure) and other serious problems associated with multiples can threaten the health of the mother.

Today's fertility specialists strive to reduce those risks by limiting the number of embryos they implant for IVF or canceling intrauterine insemination (IUI) cycles if there's a high probability of multiple gestations. Following American Society for Reproductive Medicine (ASRM) guidelines, most fertility specialists recommend transferring one to two embryos for women under age thirty-five; two to four for women ages thirty-five to forty; and three to five for women over age forty. Your doctor will discuss what's acceptable for you and may suggest deviating slightly from the guidelines if he or she thinks it's medically appropriate based on your reproductive history. With the advent of blastocyst transfer, fertility specialists can reduce the number of embryos they put back into the uterus and still be confident of good success rates.

Keep in mind, however, that, even when guidelines are followed, there's always a risk of multiples. They occur in 15 to 35 percent of women, depending on their age.

Should you fail to get pregnant on the first IVF attempt, or lose the embryo, you still may succeed in the future. If pregnancy doesn't occur on a second or third attempt, however, you'll need to look at other options, because IVF success rates drop significantly with more than three attempts. For couples who have repeated implantation failures, there are still alternatives.

Other ART Options

Gamete Intrafallopian Tube Transfer (GIFT)

The fertility treatment known as *gamete intrafallopian tube transfer* (*GIFT*) allows fertilization to occur within the body rather than in a petri dish in a lab. A woman's gametes, or eggs, are removed from the ovaries, immediately mixed with *washed sperm,* and placed back into the fallopian tube—rather than into the uterus, as done with IVF—through laparoscopy. Although GIFT is an alternative to IVF, the IVF procedure offers several advantages: It doesn't require laparoscopic techniques to place the embryos back into the woman's body; fertilization can be confirmed before implantation; and the results are generally excellent.

Zygote Intrafallopian Tube Transfer (ZIFT)

Another ART procedure, *zygote intrafallopian tube transfer* (*ZIFT*) involves uniting sperm and eggs in a laboratory and then implanting fertilized embryos inside the fallopian tube. Since this process takes place in the lab, the embryologist can verify that fertilization actually occurred prior to implantation (unlike with GIFT).

Women undergoing ZIFT experience the same preparatory steps as for IVF. However, after fertilization is confirmed, an appropriate number of day one embryos are transferred to the fallopian tube, rather than the uterus, through laparoscopy. This placement exposes the embryos to nutrients so that the early progress is more natural when they move into the uterine cavity four days later. The timing ensures that the embryos are in perfect sync with the uterus.

Although GIFT, ZIFT, and IVF produce similar outcomes, success with GIFT and ZIFT also depend on your doctor's laparoscopic skills. But if you've had repeated failures with traditional IVF, GIFT and ZIFT are options.

Embryo Genetic Testing

If your physician is concerned that your embryo is at risk for a chromosomal abnormality or gene mutation, he or she may recommend *preimplantation genetic diagnosis (PGD)*. PGD offers advantages over *amniocentesis* or *chorionic villus sampling (CVS)*, the standard genetic tests done on the amniotic fluid or placenta wall during pregnancy. By testing IVF-produced embryos before transfer, PGD eliminates other test-related risks, such as losing a fetus or facing termination of a pregnancy. Instead, it increases the chances of having a healthy baby because only normal embryos are used.

DNA, Genes, and Chromosomes

PGD can discover genetic problems caused by a variety of abnormalities involving *DNA (deoxyribonucleic acid), genes,* and *chromosomes.* Although the terms are often used interchangeably, these structures have distinctive (yet mutual) cellular functions. DNA is the genetic code, or blueprint, necessary to construct and direct each cell. It determines every unique characteristic, from eye color to blood type. Genes are the DNA segments that carry that genetic information. An estimated twenty-five thousand of them are contained in each chromosome, the organizational structure housing the DNA inside an individual cell. Every cell contains twenty-three chromosomal pairs, with each parent contributing one member, for a total of forty-six chromosomes.

Chromosomal abnormalities. Extra, missing, or fragmented chromosomes can lead to repeated failed pregnancies, miscarriages, or developmental problems such as mental retardation or heart defects. Chromosomal problems are often related to *aneuploidy,* spontaneous chromosomal damage to an older woman's aging eggs. The resulting embryos don't divide normally, or, if they do, they don't implant or survive a full-term pregnancy. Occasionally, an embryo will survive, but with major birth defects, such as Down's syndrome, caused by an extra, or third, copy of chromosome 21 (known as *Trisomy 21*).

Genetic abnormalities. Changes in chromosomes or a *single gene mutation* on a specific chromosome also may result in serious disorders, such as sickle-cell anemia or cystic fibrosis (CF). It's unclear what triggers most genetic abnormalities. Some alterations in a gene's DNA sequence appear spontaneously, while others may be linked to environmental toxins, such as radiation. Many genetic abnormalities are passed from parent to child; in some cases, it takes only one parent to have the mutated gene, while in other cases, it takes both parents to put the fetus at risk.

Deciding When to Test

Because it needs to be done in a laboratory, PGD is used only to detect genetic changes in embryos created with IVF. Embryos are allowed to develop until day three, when a single cell is extracted through a hole in the outer shell. The embryos will be checked for gene-related disorders such as the following:

- *Chromosomal abnormalities*—conditions, such as Down's syndrome, related to chromosomal additions, duplications, deletions, or rearrangements
- *Sex-, or X-, linked* disorders—conditions, such as hemophilia, related to an error on the X chromosome
- *Single gene defects*—conditions, such as Tay-Sachs disease, related to a mutation on one specific gene

There are risks to PGD testing that must be considered on an individual basis. The biopsy procedure could damage or kill the embryo—although this outcome is uncommon when the procedure is performed by an experienced embryologist. Nonetheless, because there are a finite number of inherited disorders that can be tested, PGD is usually offered only to couples with a documented familial risk of a serious or life-threatening illness being passed on to a child.

In some cases, however, fertility specialists will recommend preimplantation genetic screening (PGS) for couples presumed to be chromosomally normal but still at risk for a spontaneous abnormality, particularly because of the mother's age. Experts disagree on the role of PGS; it's not recommended routinely at this time. But if you're in your late thirties and/or you've had repeated IVF failures or pregnancy losses, your physician may suggest it.

PGD can reliably determine the sex of an embryo, but because of the potential risks involved, this use is usually discouraged. Some couples request the test to gender-balance their families, but such a controversial use raises many issues, particularly in determining what to do with embryos of the "wrong" sex. Fertility clinics often suggest that the embryos be donated anonymously to another childless couple. In any case, couples considering PGD for no other reason than to learn the sex of their embryos should be carefully counseled.

Selective Reduction

If your fertility treatment procedure has yielded triplets or *higher-order multiples*, you and your doctor may want to explore *selective reduction.* By removing some fetuses, the remaining fetuses will likely have enough room in the uterus to thrive during the pregnancy.

Selective reduction is typically performed between the eleventh and thirteenth weeks of pregnancy by a *perina-tologist*, an obstetrical specialist trained to care for high-risk fetuses. The technique has much in common with amniocentesis, in that a needle is usually inserted through the abdominal wall into the uterus; however, in this case, the needle is then inserted into the fetal heart sac. After an injection of potassium chloride stops the heart of the fetus, the woman's body absorbs the fetal material. There's no one set of criteria for choosing which fetus to terminate, although the health of the fetus and accessibility are common factors.

Sometimes, selective reduction occurs naturally during the first trimester, when a fetus simply stops growing. Because the fetus is eventually absorbed by the woman's body, it represents a small risk for the surviving fetuses.

Since selective reduction is legal in all fifty states, it's not controversial as a matter of law. But some people have moral concerns about it. Many couples are uncomfortable with the idea of selective reduction. But without selective reduction, high-order multiples face almost certain premature birth and, often, lifelong health issues.

Whatever your view, it's important that you receive all relevant information prior to undergoing selective reduction. Your doctor and perhaps a counselor can help guide you through the decision-making process.

Cryopreservation

Modern freezing techniques, known as *cryopreservation* techniques, play an important role in fertility treatment. Cryopreservation increases the likelihood of couples conceiving by making donor specimens possible and available when needed. Freezing also allows couples to preserve their own sperm, eggs, and/or extra embryos should they want to try additional treatment cycles later. Although success varies, cryopreservation can provide the means to conceive now or in the future.

Freezing Sperm

For decades, men have been able to donate or store their sperm by having it frozen. Because of cryopreservation, sperm banks across the country can provide couples immediate access to healthy sperm. The technology also allows men to preserve their own sperm for future use—which is particularly helpful if they're concerned about not being able to produce sperm in the future. This may be the case of a man who must undergo cancer treatment and has been told he won't be able to produce sperm afterward. It may also be the case for a man prior to having a vasectomy.

Cryopreservation of sperm involves several steps, starting with a semen analysis to determine if the man's sperm meets acceptable standards. Specimens may be washed or left unwashed, and are then divided into small batches, transferred into sealed, labeled vials, and the vials are immersed in a kind of "human antifreeze." The specimens are then frozen in liquid nitrogen vapor to ensure the least damage. They're eventually transferred into liquid nitrogen tanks for permanent storage at minus 396 degrees Fahrenheit. When needed, the sperm is slowly thawed and analyzed. Some studies suggest that frozen and fresh sperm fertility and live birth rates are comparable.

Freezing Eggs

Although doctors have been successfully freezing sperm for years, they haven't had the same experience with freezing eggs. Female eggs contain a great deal of water (more than sperm), which makes them susceptible to damage from razor-sharp ice crystals.

Recent research, however, has yielded new ways to protect eggs during cryopreservation. Higher concentrates of freezing fluids are now used to extract more water from the eggs. In addition, a newer, rapid freezing technique, called *vitrification*, speeds up the process. By instantaneously freezing the eggs in a liquid nitrogen bath at minus 396 degrees Fahrenheit, this technique limits crystallization. When a woman is ready to attempt another pregnancy, the egg is then thawed quickly and washed of the cryoprotectant before being inseminated through in vitro fertilization (IVF)/intracytoplasmic sperm injection (ICSI).

Although it has been approved by the FDA, vitrification remains a newer technology. Many fertility specialists are using it for targeted groups, such as young cancer patients who want to preserve their eggs prior to radiation or chemotherapy because the treatment might lead to premature ovarian failure (POF). The technique shows promise for other women, as well, particularly those interested in delaying childbearing. However, since there's not enough research to demonstrate that eggs stored longer than a few years can be successfully thawed and fertilized, women are cautioned about using cryopreservation for delaying pregnancy.

Freezing Embryos

Cryopreservation is most commonly used when couples undergoing IVF wish to freeze their extra embryos for a future pregnancy attempt. It's also useful when a woman has produced such a large number of eggs during one treatment cycle that she's at risk for ovarian hyperstimulation syndrome (OHSS). The eggs are recovered and fertilized, and the resulting embryos are frozen for implantation during a later cycle, when there's no risk of OHSS because the ovaries aren't being stimulated.

Though freezing can be done at any stage of embryo development, many doctors prefer that it be done at either day three or day five to improve pregnancy rates. The embryos are slowly cooled in a cryoprotectant fluid and then stored in either sealed vials or straws in large nitrogen tanks at minus 396 degrees Fahrenheit. When a couple is ready to attempt pregnancy, the embryos are thawed, rinsed, and placed in an incubator until transfer. Because freezing can harden the outer wall of an embryo, assisted hatching is often used to optimize implantation.

If they're of good quality, your embryos can be frozen now, thawed later, and still produce good pregnancy results. However, if they're not of good quality going into the process, they're likely to fragment or die after thawing. Also, live birth rates are lower with cryopreserved embryos than with fresh embryos. With recent FDA approval for all embryo stages, however, vitrification has promise as a more successful approach to cryopreservation than the standard "slow" freeze. There is also a concern about birth defects in children produced from frozen/thawed embryos; however, studies have shown no statistical increase in defects over the rest of the population.

One advantage to freezing embryos is that you can reduce the time and cost of subsequent pregnancy attempts, because you won't need to undergo the entire ovulation stimulation process again. Plus, if you were younger when your embryos were frozen, you'll decrease the risk of chromosomal abnormalities and miscarriage associated with being older. An additional benefit of cryopreservation is that you have the option of donating your remaining frozen embryos anonymously once you've completed your family.

Selecting a Fertility Clinic

Naturally, couples considering IVF or other procedures will want to find a clinic with a good success rate. Both the Centers for Disease Control and Prevention (CDC) and the Society for Assisted Reproductive Technology (SART), an affiliate organization of ASRM, provide recent statistics on individual fertility programs, through their Internet Web sites (www.cdc.gov/art or www.sart.org).

Every fertility clinic is required by federal law to report birth rates for various age categories to the CDC, along with frozen embryo statistics. SART members, whose ranks include more than 400 IVF programs in the United States, must submit annual data disclosing types of infertility patients; number of cycles versus outcomes; pregnancy and multiple pregnancy rates; and miscarriage and cancellation rates.

Although the SART data provide some basis of comparison, it's important to interpret all data and any other information about individual clinics with care. Since many factors can affect IVF performance, make sure you understand what's behind the numbers and terms, particularly the following:

- *Types of patients.* Some clinics are willing to accept women over age forty or women with very complicated fertility problems and low chances of success. These women can skew clinics' pregnancy rates downward. Other clinics choose patients for IVF or other ART procedures based entirely on their potential for success. This skews their numbers upward.
- *Number of embryos transferred per cycle.* Clinics vary in what they'll do for women, although ASRM guidelines recommend against transferring large numbers of embryos. You'll want to know about the practices of the clinic you're considering.
- *Success rate.* Federal law requires that clinics report IVF success rates in terms of "number of cycles" rather than "number of women." Since many women undergo more than one cycle, a clinic's success rate may be lower because of those multiple attempts. Also, cycle cancellations can affect success rate, so make sure you understand the clinic's experience ending IVF.
- *Defining pregnancy.* Because *pregnancy* doesn't always mean "live birth," you need to know how the clinic defines the term in relation to its statistics. A *biochemical pregnancy* means the pregnancy has been confirmed

through blood or urine tests, but isn't visible on ultrasound. A *clinical pregnancy* can be identified with ultrasound, but may stop growing at some point later. Since carrying a baby to full term is your goal, you'll want to focus on statistics concerning actual live birth rates per IVF cycle when comparing clinics.

Do you need to be a statistician to evaluate the performance of a fertility clinic? No—but you do need to be an informed consumer. Fertility specialists should be able to explain their per-cycle track record with live births, multiple births, miscarriages, and cancellations. Just make sure the statistics are specific to your age group.

Beyond the numbers, there are other important factors to consider in selecting an IVF program. It's always important to have a doctor with whom you feel comfortable and can communicate, particularly when you need to undergo advanced fertility treatment. Numbers alone won't tell you if a fertility specialist has the kind of personal skills and manner you're seeking. Recommendations from others who've undergone such treatments can be very helpful for this part of your search.

7

Reproductive Surgery

Not every female fertility problem can be solved with drugs or assisted reproductive technologies (ARTs). As effective as these techniques are in treating infertility, they can't take care of any physical problems that might be preventing you from getting pregnant. If you've been diagnosed with endometriosis, ovarian cysts, or fibroids, your doctor may suggest corrective surgery. If you have the surgery, you may not need further treatment. But even if you do need additional treatment, the surgery will likely improve your chances of becoming pregnant.

Finding a Skilled Surgeon

Reproductive surgeons are reproductive endocrinologists (REs) who've undergone extensive training in microsurgical, laparoscopic, and other endoscopic techniques. Not all REs are trained in reproductive surgery, and with the advent of in vitro fertilization (IVF), many fellowship programs have de-emphasized such surgery skills because doctors can facilitate conception in the laboratory. If you need gynecologic surgery, it's important to find a fertility specialist with a proven reproductive surgery record.

Surgical Procedures

Laparoscopy

As mentioned in an earlier chapter, laparoscopy is an effective tool both for diagnosing and treating fertility problems. By inserting a fiber-optic scope through the navel and manipulating other tools through small incisions, doctors can remove fibroids, ovarian cysts, benign tumors, and pelvic adhesions. They can also burn away endometrial tissue, treat tubal pregnancies, and recover eggs for gamete intrafallopian tube transfer (GIFT) or zygote intrafallopian tube transfer (ZIFT). Although doctors can't guarantee pregnancy, correcting an underlying problem through laparoscopy may pave the way.

Endometriosis. Your doctor will likely recommend laparoscopic cautery or laser vaporization to remove unwanted endometrial tissue. The technique burns away the tissue, reducing the risk of pelvic damage or adhesions. If you have residual endometriosis following laparoscopy, your doctor may want to shrink the remaining tissue by starving it of hormonal stimulation with leuprolide acetate (Lupron), a gonadotropin-releasing hormone (GnRH) agonist.

Even if you have extensive endometriosis, there's no reason to end all hopes of pregnancy by having a hysterectomy (removal of the uterus), as is sometimes recommended. With today's surgical and medical approaches, doctors can eliminate the excess tissue, likely allowing you to conceive.

Ovarian cysts and benign tumors. Not all ovarian cysts need treatment, but those that do usually can be removed effectively with laparoscopy. The procedure may allow your doctor to save the ovary. Similarly, benign ovarian tumors can be eliminated with laparoscopy. Since these masses grow bigger over time and can crush the surrounding ovarian tissue, it's best if your doctor removes them early on. In both cases, the procedure may allow your doctor to save the ovary.

Hysteroscopy

Like laparoscopy, hysteroscopy is an effective option for diagnosing and treating uterine growths and other uterine abnormalities. With the hysteroscope inserted through the cervix into the uterine cavity, your doctor can simultaneously view and cut away fibroids and polyps with a rotating blade. This technology has made a profound difference in reproductive surgery over the past several years by reducing both operating time and tissue injury. Because growths can be removed without burning them or introducing electrical energy into the uterine cavity, the chance of injuring the surrounding tissues is greatly reduced.

Uterine fibroids. Many women with fibroids can get pregnant and carry a baby to full term. In some cases, however, the growths can prevent conception and increase the risk of miscarriage. Doctors are most concerned about large single fibroids or clusters of fibroids, especially those that arise within the uterine cavity.

Although fertility specialists sometimes recommend medication to shrink fibroids, the growths can return once treatment is stopped and/or when a woman becomes pregnant. If they return when you're pregnant, they can cause other complications. In severe cases, doctors often recommend hyster-ectomy; however, a physician skilled in hysteroscopy can eliminate even large, partially embedded growths, with minimal tissue damage, thus preserving your hopes of having a baby.

Septate and bicornuate uteri. A septate uterus is a birth defect in which a band of fibrous tissue divides the uterine cavity in half. Another birth defect, a bicornuate uterus has protrusions at the top of either side of it, sometimes giving the uterus a distinct heart shape. Both these conditions can lead to pregnancy loss.

Unlike some uterine defects, a septate or bicornuate uterus can be fixed surgically, if necessary. If you have a septate uterus, your doctor will likely suggest hysteroscopy with laparoscopy. If your diagnosis is a bicornuate uterus, surgery is usually best performed via *laparotomy* (working through an abdominal incision), rather than laparoscopy (working through the navel). Because some women with these conditions don't miscarry, doctors sometimes suggest attempting pregnancy before having surgery. However, since there's no way to predict who will be successful, unifying the uterus first may be the best approach.

Microsurgery

Performed using specialized instruments under an operating microscope, microsurgery involves handling tissue delicately so there's minimal damage to it. Microsurgery is used primarily to unblock the fallopian tubes and to reverse tubal ligation. By magnifying the area five to forty times, a microscope allows a reproductive surgeon to work on structures barely visible to the naked eye. Also, because the surrounding tissue is kept moist and bleeding is minimized, the risk of developing scar tissue is reduced.

Tubal ligation is reversed by reconnecting the tiny ends of the fallopian tubes with extremely small sutures. As long as the remaining sections are of sufficient length, a skilled reproductive surgeon can reconnect them. In most cases, no matter how your tubal ligation was performed (through cutting, tying, clamping, or burning), the tubes can be reopened to stay open.

Some doctors suggest bypassing the tubes altogether and using IVF instead. But you should be aware of the pros and cons of both procedures. IVF will likely produce a pregnancy, but you may have to undergo several attempts, each one more expensive than surgery. Surgery involves minimal risk and a short recovery, and once your tubes are reconnected, you have a good chance of becoming pregnant without further treatment. Pregnancy rates with this procedure are between 50 and 70 percent, depending on a woman's age, and women in their forties may conceive. The average time to pregnancy is six to seven months.

8

Male Infertility

Unlike female infertility, which can involve many problems, male infertility involves just one: sperm. If a man can't produce and deliver enough quality sperm, he can't impregnate his partner. Fortunately, medical science has identified impediments to normal sperm production and delivery. And with today's technologies, doctors can diagnose and overcome most of those impediments.

Before examining the causes of male infertility, let's review the basics of the male reproductive system.

The Basics of Male Reproduction

The focus of reproduction in men is on the testicles, where sperm originates and matures. But the penis is also essential for ejaculation and delivery of sperm. Other glands, organs, and hormonal signals from the brain play a role, too.

Testicles

The testicles, or testes, are the center of sperm production. These paired glands form in the abdomen during a male's embryonic development, gradually descending into a skin pouch called the *scrotum*. The scrotum protects the testicles and keeps them at an optimal temperature (2 degrees below body temperature) for sperm production. Structures involved in the production of sperm include:

- *seminiferous tubules*—the delicate coils where sperm is produced.

- *epididymis*—the tightly bound tube behind the testicles, where sperm matures.
- *seminal vesicles* and *prostate*—glands that secrete 95 percent of the fluids necessary to transport sperm into the vagina and buffer its acidity.
- *vas deferens*—the cordlike duct on each side of the testicles that connects the epididymis to the penis. The ducts also carry the seminal and prostatic fluids necessary to transport sperm for ejaculation.

Male Reproductive System

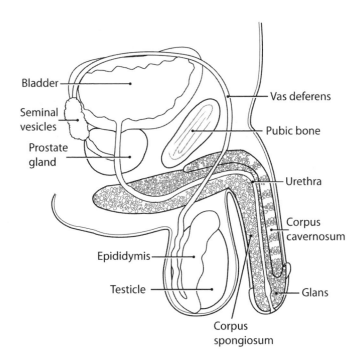

Penis

The penis is the sex organ that allows a man to deposit his sperm inside his partner's vagina. Intercourse is made possible when the spongy tissues of the penis engorge with blood, causing the penis to become erect. The inability to sustain an erection, known as erectile dysfunction, can be a factor in a man's ability to impregnate a woman. Incidentally, penis size has little or no bearing on a man's ability to produce and deliver sperm. As long as a penis can deliver sperm near the cervix, size is rarely an issue.

Sperm

Men produce millions of new sperm every day. They're constantly replenishing their supply, even into their sixties and seventies. Each sperm is microscopically tiny, but very complex, with three distinct parts: the head, which contains genetic material (DNA); the midpiece, which contains energizing fructose; and the tail, which propels the sperm forward with the help of semen, the fluid portion of a man's ejaculate. Semen is composed of secretions from the *seminal vesicles* and the *prostate*. It not only transports sperm and buffers the acidity of the vagina, but also provides nutrients to keep sperm healthy.

It's true that making a baby takes only one sperm. However, for natural conception to occur, hundreds of millions of sperm are needed initially so that enough healthy ones survive the journey to the fallopian tubes, where one sperm can join with an egg. What happens to the rest of them? Millions may be lost in the ejaculate that normally spills out after intercourse. Millions more may be filtered out by the acidity of the vagina and cervical mucus. Of the remaining sperm that travel through the uterus, a select group of two hundred to three hundred swim up the fallopian tubes and "compete" to impregnate a woman's egg.

Hormones

The male reproductive system would not function properly without follicle-stimulating hormone (FSH) and luteinizing hormone (LH). These hormones perform the same "stimulating" role in men as they do in women. LH also prompts the *Leydig cells* within the testicles to produce *testosterone*, the primary male sex hormone.

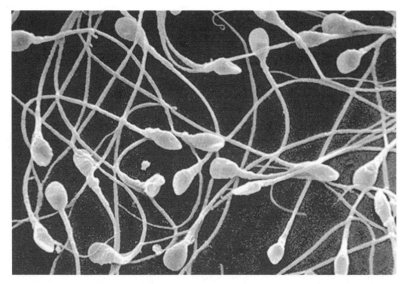

Male sperm magnified one thousand times. *Photo: PhototakeUSA*

Causes of Male Infertility

Problems with Sperm

For many years, fertility specialists thought that the amount of sperm in a man's ejaculate was *the* critical factor in conception. In fact, decreased sperm count does make impregnating a partner more difficult—but not impossible. And although sperm count is critical, doctors have learned that *motility* (movement) and *morphology* (appearance) are just as important. In fact, the chances of achieving pregnancy improve if at least half of the man's sperm have good function, shape, and size. Under the microscope, a healthy sperm looks much like a needle in motion. It has a smooth, oval-shaped head, with no defects in the neck or midpiece and a tail that swishes to propel it forward.

The closer a man is to ideal "sperm parameters," the greater his likelihood of impregnating a woman through intercourse. Conversely, the further away his sperm count, motility, and morphology are from ideal, the more help he'll need in getting his sperm to the egg. The volume of semen is also important, since semen transports the sperm and also provides nutrients to keep sperm healthy. (Typically, men generate between 2 and 5 milliliters, or up to a teaspoonful, of seminal fluid every time they ejaculate.)

Although sperm problems vary, there are two basic categories at the heart of most male fertility problems: *oligospermia*, which is a sperm count of less than 20 million/milliliter, and *azoospermia*, which is a sperm count of zero. A sperm count of zero means a man is sterile.

What causes a low sperm count or no sperm? In 90-plus percent of cases, the underlying problem is *idiopathic*, or unknown. In other cases, however, a low sperm count or no sperm can be traced to very specific causes: swollen scrotal veins; infections; hormone imbalances; immunological, chromosomal, or congenital disorders; medications; supplements such as *anabolic steroids* and *human growth hormone* (*hGH*); duct system damage; ejaculatory malfunctions; and alcohol and marijuana. (There's no merit to the popular myths that tight underwear, hot tubs, and too much sex reduce sperm count.) Whether these problems impede sperm production or delivery, the outcome is the same: sperm too diminished to impregnate.

Varicoceles

Commonly called "varicose veins of the testicles," a *varicoceles* is a snakelike bundle of abnormally swollen blood vessels in the scrotum. They form when a defective valve, which would normally usher blood away from the testicles toward the abdomen, fails to close, leaving the blood to pool in the scrotum. The condition can affect one or both testicles.

An estimated 40 to 50 percent of men with fertility problems have detectable varicoceles. However, because varicoceles are often found in men with normal fertility, the association with infertility remains vague. A primary theory is that accumulated blood in the scrotum raises the temperature around the testicles, slowing or reducing sperm production. Often the first symptom of the condition, impaired semen quality may also be a factor.

A varicocele diagnosis is made through a physical examination and ultrasound. In addition to swelling in the scrotum, a visible sign of the condition is an atrophied testicle on the same side as the bundle of swollen veins.

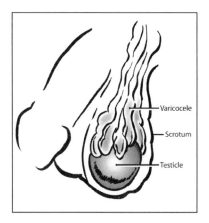

A varicocele is a bundle of swollen blood vessels in the scrotum, most commonly found on the left testicle. It can cause low sperm production.

Infections

Infections can affect male fertility by reducing sperm production and movement or by causing scarring that blocks sperm passage. The most common culprit is mumps, which can result in *orchitis,* a condition of the testicles involving inflammation, swelling, and/or frequent infections. Although mumps is usually a childhood disease, if the disease is contracted after puberty, the virus can settle in the testicles, eventually disrupting sperm production.

Testicular swelling also can occur as a symptom of other infections that may affect sperm production or delivery. These infections include *prostatitis,* or inflammation of the prostate; *epididymitis,* or inflammation of the epididymis; and Chlamydia. If left untreated, Chlamydia infection can cause *urethritis,* inflammation of the urethra, the duct that carries sperm, semen, and urine through the penis.

Infections that might have a bearing on fertility are usually screened with urine tests, although the gold standard is a urethral swab culture. These infections are generally treated with antibiotics. Fertility treatment will be delayed until the infection is brought under control, which may take several months.

Hormone Deficiencies

As mentioned earlier, some of the same hormones that play an essential role in female reproduction also play a role in male reproduction. A man's pituitary gland releases FSH and LH, starting a cascade of events leading to sperm production. In particular, LH stimulates specialized testicular cells, called Leydig cells, to make the male hormone testosterone. Although rare in relation to other factors, hormone deficiencies can hinder sperm production enough to cause fertility problems.

Men with particularly low levels of FSH and LH are sometimes diagnosed with *hypogonadotropic hypogonadism,* or severe underactivity of the testes. The condition results in a variety of male sexual deficiencies, including reduced sperm production. Hormone problems are usually diagnosed with standard blood tests. However, if the doctor suspects hypogonadotropic hypogonadism, he or she may order chromosomal and other tests, since the condition can be caused by problems other than hormone deficiencies. As long as there are no underlying problems, sperm production can be restored by treatment with supplemental FSH and LH.

Immunological Disorders

Immunological problems involve the body attacking its own cells as if they're viruses or bacteria. About 10 percent of men with fertility problems are believed to produce "direct" antisperm antibodies (ASAs), special proteins that interfere with the sperm's motility and ability to penetrate a woman's egg. Antisperm antibodies are extremely uncommon, except in males with a history of testicular injury, trauma, or surgery.

ASAs are most often suspected when a man has had a vasectomy and a vasectomy reversal. When the vas deferens (the tubes that carry sperm from the scrotum to the urethra) are cut, sperm can be released into the bloodstream. Because the immune system doesn't recognize the sperm as belonging there, it makes antibodies against them. The antibodies are generally of no consequence until a man decides to reverse the surgery. By then, the antibodies have passed throughout the testicles. Even if a vasectomy reversal results in sperm in the ejaculate, the antibodies may attach to the sperm, preventing them from moving and fertilizing an egg.

Because doctors know who's at risk for ASAs, they also know whom to target. Antisperm antibodies are confirmed through a blood or semen test. Some physicians treat the disorder with low-dose prednisone.

Chromosomal Disorders

Chromosomal problems can also affect sperm production. Five to 10 percent of men with either low sperm counts or no sperm suffer from a Y chromosome abnormality, a genetic defect that prevents normal sperm development. The most severe abnormality is *Sertoli cell-only syndrome*, a rare condition in which sperm-producing cells never formed in the testicles during fetal development.

Klinefelter's syndrome occurs in men who have an extra X chromosome in addition to their XY chromosomes (for example, XXY). This condition can cause higher-than-normal FSH and LH levels, resulting in a lower-than-normal testosterone level. Although decreased facial and body hair is an indicator of Klinefelter's, the bigger problems are smaller testicles and a sperm count that is low or at zero.

Chromosomal abnormalities are diagnosed with blood tests. Since these genetic factors can't be changed, the best treatment will be in vitro fertilization (IVF) and/or the use of donor sperm, depending on the results of the semen analysis.

Congenital Disorders

No sperm or a persistently low sperm count (20 million/milliliter or less) can also result when a part of the reproductive system is either malformed or missing. An *undescended testicle*, for example, is an uncommon disorder in which a testicle develops normally in the abdomen but fails to drop into the scrotum prior to birth. Being diagnosed with this problem doesn't mean that a man can't father a child. But unless his testicle is surgically repositioned (before age six), impregnating a partner later in life will be difficult, due to a markedly reduced sperm count. In this case, IVF may be required for his partner to achieve pregnancy.

Some men are born without a vas deferens. This problem is often symptomatic of an underlying genetic condition, particularly cystic fibrosis (CF). Although CF is a serious disease marked by abnormal, sticky mucus in the lungs, sometimes the symptoms are so mild that it goes undetected. If CF is suspected, the doctor will likely suggest genetic screening before fertility treatment, since the disease can be passed on. Doctors use ultrasound and other imaging tests to diagnose a missing vas deferens. Fertility treatment in this case involves recovering sperm from the testicle and joining it with a woman's egg via IVF/intracytoplasmic sperm injection (ICSI).

Medications

Some medications can interfere with sperm production or delivery. For example, *antibiotics* and *antifungals* can interfere with sperm production, and certain drugs used to treat high blood pressure (*antihypertensives*) and depression (*antidepressants*) are known to cause problems with erection. Doctors may recommend switching medications or discontinuing them during fertility treatment, depending on a man's reliance on the medication and his overall health.

Anabolic steroids, such as testosterone and human growth hormone (hGH), and other body-building supplements can also cause problems with male fertility. They can suppress a man's hormones, causing his testicles to shrink (sometimes to the size of raisins) and lowering his sperm count. Although the damage can be permanent with long-term use, it is usually reversed if the supplements are stopped early enough.

Prior Vasectomy and Damage to Ducts

Of course, even if a man has had a vasectomy, he is still able to produce sperm. A vasectomy involves surgically cutting the vasa deferentia to prevent the delivery of sperm. Since a vasectomy doesn't prevent the prostate and other glands from secreting seminal fluids, there's little effect on the volume of a man's ejaculate.

Men with fertility problems can experience blockages in any part of the ductal system: the epididymis, vasa deferentia, and *ejaculatory ducts*. The obstructions may be congenital, or they can occur later in life. A hernia repair, for instance, can damage the vas deferens, causing a blockage and affecting sperm production. Ductal problems are diagnosed with imaging tests.

Ejaculatory Problems

Among the ejaculatory factors that can impede sperm delivery, impotence is easily the most identifiable. No matter how good a man's sperm may be, he can't father a child through normal intercourse if he can't achieve or maintain an erection. Although low self-esteem, performance anxiety, and other psychological issues can be factors in impotence, physical problems can be the source of the problem. Men suffering from diabetes, heart disease, or high blood pressure often have erection problems because of diminished blood flow to the penis. Antidepressants and other medications can also cause erection problems.

Among other delivery problems associated with male infertility, *retrograde ejaculation* is perhaps the most common. It occurs when a man's seminal fluid flows backward into the bladder instead of propelling forward through the penis during orgasm. Retrograde ejaculation occurs because the sphincter, the muscle that normally opens and closes the bladder, fails to close properly, allowing semen to be thrust into the bladder during intercourse. Retrograde ejaculation can be caused by blood pressure medications or medical problems such as diabetes, prostate surgery, and spinal cord injury. Doctors will suspect retrograde ejaculation if a man's urine is milky. Another sign is a semen analysis that shows little or no seminal fluid.

Getting a Diagnosis

Investigating male infertility requires the same methodical diagnostic approach that's used with females. Because male infertility involves the urinary tract, a *urologist* is often involved in the initial exam and later if surgery is required. A urologist has completed medical school plus a five-year residency focused on the evaluation and treatment of disorders of the kidneys, urinary tract, bladder, and male reproductive organs.

If a couple is working with a gynecologist or primary care physician, the doctor often will refer the man to a urologist immediately in order to check semen and sperm, hormone levels, and for any physical problems. But if the couple is already working with a reproductive endocrinologist (RE), the more likely scenario is that the RE will do the initial testing and consult a urologist if there's a problem that needs further investigation. The ideal scenario is for these physicians to coordinate tests and plot treatment as a team.

History/Physical Examination/Testing

Because male factors are involved in so many infertility cases, a fertility specialist will want a complete picture of a man's health before moving forward with fertility treatment. Most doctors prefer to order a semen/sperm analysis on the man at the same time that they're performing blood and other initial tests on the woman. Although abnormal results in men often have no known cause, the doctor will still want to review the man's medical history and perform a physical examination.

The doctor will likely be interested in the man's past sexual problems, frequency of intercourse, and success at fathering children. He or she will also want to know about:

- past or recent infections or a high fever within the past three months
- past illnesses or diseases or a family history of diseases such as cystic fibrosis
- past surgeries, such as a vasectomy or a bladder or hernia repair
- past injury or trauma to the testicles
- the presence of varicoceles (swollen scrotal veins) or other testicular swelling
- congenital abnormalities
- current medications, particularly antihypertensives and antidepressants
- use of anabolic steroids, such as testosterone or hGH

- alcohol, cocaine, marijuana, or nicotine use
- any exposure to potential occupational or environmental toxins

In addition to taking a history, the doctor may send the man to a urologist for a thorough physical examination, particularly of the penis, testicles, prostate, and scrotum. He or she will want to know, for instance, if the testicles and the network of tubes surrounding them are the correct sizes and in the correct locations. Since 95 percent of a testicle is comprised of sperm-producing cells, small testicles usually indicate a significant reduction in sperm production. The doctor will also check for varicoceles. These abnormal swellings can usually be detected by manipulating the scrotum with the fingers.

There are many subsequent tests a doctor could perform, but the most likely ones include:

- blood tests to reveal abnormal levels of the hormones FSH, LH, testosterone, or prolactin, possibly indicating endocrine or testicular problems
- additional blood tests to detect other medical problems, such as an infection
- ultrasound and other imaging techniques to view the interior reproductive structures, to detect or verify varicoceles, duct obstructions, or other abnormalities

Although the results of these tests may be helpful in uncovering a potential cause, physicians frequently can make a diagnosis of male infertility based on a medical history, an examination, and the all-important semen analysis.

Semen Analysis

A semen analysis should be a routine part of every initial fertility evaluation. A semen analysis is a fairly inexpensive tool for the valuable information it yields: data on semen volume and sperm count, motility, and morphology.

Many men find semen collection an embarrassing, intrusive task because it needs to be done in a specific way, using a specific timeline, to ensure the accuracy and validity of a semen analysis. Prior to collection, the man will have to refrain from ejaculating for two to five days to optimize the number of sperm in the sample. To collect the semen, the man is asked to masturbate and catch his ejaculate in a sterile container. Doctors usually prefer that this be done in the office so that the sample can be delivered to the lab in a timely manner. An office collection also ensures that the fluid remains at body temperature. Some clinics allow men to collect their semen at home and place it in a thermos, but they must get it to the lab within sixty minutes of ejaculating, to guarantee viability.

The doctor may need more than one specimen in order to obtain accurate data. Since it takes the testicles three months to make new sperm, ejaculate on any given day could be affected by previous fevers, viruses, infections, medications, or other factors such as alcohol, marijuana, or steroid use. For that reason, doctors often prefer to obtain several samples at specific intervals.

Evaluating the Specimen

Semen and sperm are evaluated using two sets of criteria: World Health Organization (WHO) standards and Kruger's Strict Morphology, so-named for its physician-developer, Thinus F. Kruger. Both approaches require immobilizing sperm on a microscopic grid to assess various features. The Kruger test, however, is considered the more sophisticated and stringent tool in assessing morphology. Because it catches the subtle, but clinically important, abnormalities often missed by WHO standards, the Kruger test is very desirable, especially prior to IVF.

Although many fertility specialists believe the Kruger test should be performed for an initial semen analysis in order to make the best recommendations, other physicians feel it's less necessary for routine sperm testing. For example, WHO criteria are usually satisfactory for decisions involving intrauterine insemination (IUI). The WHO analysis includes the following:

- *Semen volume.* Men should generate from 2 to 5 milliliters, or about a teaspoonful, of semen every time they ejaculate. Less than 2 milliliters is considered too low a volume to protect the sperm. More than 5 milliliters doesn't guarantee fertility, however. Even if a man produces twice the normal volume of semen, he can still have other problems.

- *Semen liquefaction or viscosity.* Semen coagulates like a gel immediately after ejaculation, but it should liquefy within an hour. If semen remains viscous (thick), it's difficult for sperm to swim out of it and into the cervical mucus to fertilize an egg. Semen is evaluated to see if it remains gelled within that first hour of collection.
- *Sperm concentration, or density, within the semen.* A good sperm count is critical to conception. The concentration, or density, is measured by examining a man's semen under a microscope to see how many sperm, immobilized by a special water solution, appear within the squares of a grid pattern. The technician counts the number of sperm over several grids and multiplies that number by 1 million. The process is then repeated, and the totals averaged. Sperm count is considered normal if the density in the ejaculate is greater than 20 million/milliliter or at least 40 million sperm per ejaculate.
- *Sperm motility.* To assess sperm movement, the percentage of moving sperm in ten random microscopic fields is measured within two to three hours of ejaculation. Normal motility means that more than 40 percent of the sperm are alive, moving actively, and advancing. Forward progression is graded on a scale of one or two as fair to poor, and three or four as good to excellent. Fast, forward-moving sperm have the best chance of fertilizing an egg.
- *Sperm morphology.* Although doctors once believed that sperm count was the most important factor in getting a woman pregnant, they now believe that sperm function and appearance (such as shape and size) are just as important. Even if a man's sperm count is low, his chances of impregnating a woman improve if at least half his sperm have good function and morphology.

To determine morphology with the Kruger test, a sterile slide is smeared with freshly ejaculated semen. The semen is then air-dried and stained with a special product before being magnified one thousand times under a microscope. About one hundred sperm are evaluated for size, shape, and defects or irregularities. Normal sperm exhibit very specific anatomical features:

- a mature, oval-shaped head with smooth contours and a well-defined "cap" taking up 40 to 70 percent of the head
- no visible defects in the neck or midpiece
- a tail that can't be bent or coiled

A man has an excellent prognosis for fertilizing an egg on his own if 15 percent or more of his sperm are identified as normal. If the number is between 5 and 14 percent, his prospects range from fair to good. For men with numbers below 4 percent, the prognosis is very poor, and the use of assisted reproductive technologies (ARTs) will likely be required.

Although many labs perform semen analysis with WHO standards, evaluating morphology with Kruger criteria requires expertise only available in a certified facility, usually connected to a fertility clinic. If your doctor uses an outside lab, you may want to ask whether it's a reputable, certified lab with quality controls and acceptable results.

9

Treatment for Male Infertility

Once diagnosed, many underlying causes of male infertility can be addressed with medication, surgery, or other treatments. But the corrections don't always lead to better "sperm parameters" or higher pregnancy rates. Fortunately, today's assisted reproductive technologies (ARTs) have made it easier for a man to overcome male infertility. With these high-tech procedures, a doctor can fertilize a woman's egg with her partner's sperm as long as both structures have reproductive potential.

Overcoming Sperm Problems

Fertility specialists have such effective ways to overcome most sperm production and delivery problems that they prefer to refer to a man who needs treatment as "subfertile" rather than "infertile." By extracting sperm and uniting it with a woman's eggs through assisted reproductive technologies, doctors can bypass most sperm problems.

Harvesting Sperm

Urologists have several ways of harvesting, or extracting, sperm. A urologist will likely choose one of the following outpatient procedures, which are usually performed with local anesthesia.

Microsurgical Epididymal Sperm Aspiration (MESA)

Microsurgical epididymal sperm aspiration (MESA) involves retrieving sperm from the epididymis. After administering local anesthesia, the urologist makes a small incision in the scrotum. He or she isolates and dilates the epididymal tubes and then withdraws fluid to be examined for sperm. MESA-harvested sperm offers several advantages, particularly for men who've had vasectomies or were born with a vas deferens missing. Because the sperm is drawn from the epididymis, the sample yields high quantities of older, more motile sperm. Many embryologists prefer MESA specimens because it is easier to separate out the quality sperm, since they're moving. There's also an abundance to freeze for subsequent in vitro fertilization (IVF) treatments.

Percutaneous Epididymal Sperm Aspiration (PESA)

With this method, the urologist retrieves sperm from the epididymis after penetrating the scrotal skin with a needle. *Percutaneous epididymal sperm aspiration (PESA)* is a less costly treatment that can be done without anesthesia, a surgical incision, or microsurgical expertise. But because it doesn't always yield sperm, PESA has largely been replaced by MESA.

Testicular Sperm Aspiration (TESA)

To perform *testicular sperm aspiration (TESA)* the physician gently inserts a needle directly into the testicle and withdraws testicular tissue; this tissue contains sperm. The procedure is performed under local anesthesia. Although sperm retrieved from the testicles is younger and less motile than epididymal sperm, it's still very viable for IVF. Like MESA, this procedure is a good option for men who don't want to reverse a vasectomy but still want to father a child. It also yields enough sperm so that some of it can be saved in a sperm bank. Choosing between MESA and TESA is often based on doctor and patient preferences; however, the choice is also reliant on the presence of sperm in the epididymis.

Testicular Biopsy

Once the sole method of determining if a man's testicles are producing sufficient sperm, a *testicular biopsy* involves using local anesthesia and making a small incision in the scrotum and removing a tissue sample for microscopic evaluation. The major advantage of a biopsy over TESA is that more sperm can be obtained, which is especially helpful for men with very low sperm counts. This procedure is also useful in determining whether a man with zero sperm in his ejaculate actually has sperm in his testicles—making it possible to pursue IVF and intracytoplasmic sperm injection (ICSI). With the advent of TESA, testicular biopsies have more limited use.

Once the sperm is harvested through any of these procedures, it can be used in any of the various forms of fertility treatment discussed in previous chapters.

Treating Other Problems

Varicoceles

Surgically eliminating the swollen veins around the testicles is a relatively common treatment for varicoceles. During an outpatient *varicocelectomy*, a urologist makes an incision in the lower abdomen or groin. After lifting the *spermatic cords* (a collection of layered tissues and bundled fibers between the abdomen and each testicle) out of the scrotum, the urologist ties off the veins.

Many fertility specialists don't recommend surgically repairing a varicocele for infertility purposes alone, because the procedure doesn't improve semen quality enough to change the ultimate fertility treatment choice. Although a number of scientific studies suggest a varicocelectomy improves sperm parameters, other large trials don't consistently reflect better pregnancy rates. So unless the repair is a man's choice or the vein is so large that it should be removed, the man can proceed to intrauterine insemination (IUI) or IVF/ICSI without surgery.

Hormone Imbalances

Abnormal hormone levels in men are often treated with the same fertility drugs taken by women: clomiphene citrate, human menopausal gonadotropin (hMG), and human chorionic gonadotropin (hCG). Although some fertility clinics recommend a daily clomiphene citrate regimen to spur testosterone into increasing sperm production, there's little consistent evidence that the medication improves sperm parameters or pregnancy rates. Doctors might offer the option, however, since a small percentage of men do respond to this drug treatment. If prescribed, the regimen must be continued for at least three months, since it takes that long for sperm to develop and gain motility. Still, because there's a very small chance of significant improvement, most men proceed immediately with IUI or IVF/ICSI.

Immunological Disorders

Antisperm antibodies (ASAs) are sometimes treated with low-dose corticosteroids, such as prednisone. But reducing the antibodies to a level that makes sperm usable for conception through intercourse isn't always successful. Since prednisone can cause complications, keeping a man on it long enough to see if the antibody count goes down and the sperm count goes up can be problematic. Still, the regimen is sometimes suggested as a first-step treatment, particularly in men who've had a vasectomy reversal and are still unable to impregnate their partner. Depending on the results, the doctor may suggest IUI, which involves placing the sperm directly into the uterus. IVF/ICSI is considered the best option, however, since one quality sperm is injected directly into an egg; the embryo is then placed into the uterus.

If a man is considering a vasectomy reversal, he should have his blood tested for antisperm antibodies. Why? If ASAs bind to more than 40 percent of his sperm, he may undergo a successful reversal but his sperm will still be nonmotile—in short, it won't move well enough to achieve a pregnancy. In that case, it is usually better for the woman to undergo IVF than for the man to undergo surgery to reverse the vasectomy. If, however, ASAs bind to less than 40 percent of the sperm, a reversal may yield a pregnancy, without IVF.

Ductal Damage

A vasectomy reversal is probably the most common male ductal repair. Usually performed by a urologist, this microsurgical procedure involves cutting away the blocked tissue and reconnecting the vasa deferentia. The major advantage of vasectomy reversal is that a couple can attempt conception with intercourse. Some statistics suggest normal sperm counts within a year in 80 percent of men, and successful pregnancies in 50 to 60 percent of cases.

Success, however, depends on various factors: the expertise of the urologist, the amount of the vasa deferentia available to reconnect, and the time elapsed since the vasectomy. The older the original procedure, the lower the sperm count after a reversal. Although oral fertility medications are sometimes used to increase sperm production, they're usually ineffective. In most cases, the best way to achieve pregnancy is with IVF/ICSI. Even with low parameters, the sperm can still successfully fertilize an egg.

Similarly, surgical repair of other ductal blockages may or may not improve sperm count. If the sole purpose of the surgery is to achieve conception, it may be better to avoid surgery (and a lengthy recovery) and proceed directly to IVF/ICSI. As long as sperm can be retrieved, there's no need for surgery.

Retrograde Ejaculation

The first line of treatment for retrograde ejaculation is often over-the-counter *pseudoephedrine (Sudafed)*. Usually used to treat cold symptoms, pseudoephedrine can be helpful in increasing the bladder neck's muscle tone, which helps the sphincter close. If there's permanent nerve damage, however, the best option is to capture the semen from a man's urine after he voids or with a catheter inserted into the bladder. The fluids are spun to separate sperm concentrate. Depending on the sperm count, IUI or IVF will be used.

10

Donor Sperm

Naturally, most couples would prefer to have a child created from their own genetic materials. But what if that's not possible? Years ago, you may have turned immediately to adoption, but with today's technology, you have other options. In vitro fertilization has made it possible for couples to conceive with donor sperm, donor eggs, and donor embryos. Perhaps these choices are not the way you envisioned a pregnancy, but they're an acceptable, maybe even a necessary, way to achieve it.

When to Consider Donor Sperm

When surgical procedures or medication regimens don't improve the quality or availability of your partner's sperm, you may wish to turn to a centuries-old concept: sperm donation. Even in Biblical times, if a Jewish man died without heirs, his brother was obligated to marry his widow and father children to carry on his name. Obviously, donor insemination is much more complicated than that, but the concept of creating a family using another man's sperm is an ancient tradition with very modern applications.

If you're a single woman with no one to father your child or in a same-sex relationship, you definitely need a sperm donor. For most couples, however, the need is prompted by a problem with the male partner. Men may have problems such as poor sperm quality, genetic disorders, congenital defects of the reproductive system, or damage to the reproductive system as a result of injury.

Choosing a Sperm Donor

Donor sperm can be from someone you know or someone you don't know. How do you make the choice?

Known Donors

Having a male friend or family member donate sperm may sound like a logical idea. However, a known donor cannot simply walk into a fertility clinic and donate sperm. He must undergo the same structured testing process as an unknown donor, including Food and Drug Administration (FDA) testing, quarantine, and other screening. Your doctor is obligated to ensure that the donor is healthy and free of infectious diseases.

In addition, in many states, known donor fathers are considered legally responsible for the child. That could mean the donor could be sued for financial support, either by you or your child (at legal age). What if your child's genetic father wants that responsibility, along with an active role in the child's life later on? Unless you're confident that your known donor will view your son or daughter as just another nephew, niece, or friend's child, the arrangement could backfire.

Unknown Donors

The vast majority of couples who need to use third-party sperm have never met the donor. They have a description of his physical characteristics, ethnicity, education, personality, temperament, hobbies, and even philosophy of life. They may even have listened to his voice on an audiotape, read his essay about his family, or studied his baby picture. But for all intents and purposes, he's anonymous. Couples use unknown donors for many reasons:

- *Availability.* You don't have to wait for a friend or family member to volunteer, because sperm banks offer immediate access to candidates.
- *Selection.* By choosing from a donor pool, you can select the characteristics that matter to you.
- *FDA testing.* You don't have to go through the expense and inconvenience of this testing, including the

six-month quarantine of the sperm and mandatory retesting of the donor, because it's already been done. The sperm is ready to use.

- *Legalities.* The very nature of anonymous sperm donation guarantees that you don't have to worry about a genetic father later wanting parental rights. There are no strings attached.

For all these reasons, many fertility specialists prefer to work with unknown donors. But how do you choose the right donor? Start by dealing with a reputable and responsible sperm bank that does the necessary screening and evaluations to ensure that donors are physically and psychologically healthy. Your fertility clinic may have its own sperm donation program; if not, your doctor can put you in touch with one that he or she trusts.

The larger the donor roster, the more likely you are to find someone with similar racial, ethnic, and other personal characteristics. Also, to accommodate children who want to know about their genetic parent in the future, today's sperm banks often provide:

- pools of donors willing to make their identity known to offspring at age eighteen
- registries to facilitate children from the same donor meeting their half-siblings
- data banks that allow children to learn more about their genetic fathers without actually meeting them

It's important that the donor program be scrupulous in its practices and extremely selective in its donors. The best programs approve as few as 1 percent (or ten in one thousand) of prospective candidates, which should reassure you that they're screening very carefully.

Screening Sperm Donors

If you need donated sperm, you'll have many sperm banks from across the country from which to choose. Keep in mind, though, that not all sperm banks have the same standards.

Although states require licensure of sperm banks, criteria differ. There's also no mandatory national accreditation or centralized certification for sperm donor banks.

The American Association of Tissue Banks (AATB), an oversight organization for organ and tissue transplant safety, offers accreditation to sperm banks. In applying for accreditation, sperm banks must submit to comprehensive on-site inspections to determine if they're professionally managed, appropriately staffed, and have policies and procedures to ensure consistent quality of care. To date, only a few U.S. sperm banks have undergone this stringent process.

Nonetheless, there are more donor controls in place today. Ever since human immunodeficiency virus (HIV), acquired immune deficiency syndrome (AIDS), and hepatitis C emerged in the 1980s as major public health threats, reputable programs have tightened their practices for screening donors, processing specimens, and policing procedures. Before these infectious diseases posed such a threat, donor insemination was performed largely with fresh sperm collected from a man selected by a fertility clinic.

Changes to that process didn't occur overnight. But the potential danger of any donor passing along a new infection, not to mention sexually transmitted diseases (STDs), prompted the FDA to establish new regulations to better protect gamete, as well as other tissue and organ, recipients. In addition, the American Society for Reproductive Medicine (ASRM) instituted parallel guidelines to help fertility clinics improve their practices—and those guidelines have impacted on sperm banks, too. Together, the safeguards have virtually eliminated the use of fresh sperm, in favor of frozen and quarantined sperm and/or semen, to ensure a safe exchange.

The FDA now mandates that sperm donors undergo testing for STDs and other infectious diseases such as rubella (German measles), syphilis, hepatitis B, hepatitis C, and HIV. Donors are also tested for *cytomegalovirus* (*CMV*), a member of the same herpes virus family that causes chicken pox. (A positive CMV result doesn't necessarily exclude someone from donating; the sperm may be matched with a positive egg donor.)

In addition to doing this testing, many sperm banks have tightened their policies about screening prospective donors, matching them to recipient couples, monitoring the donors' health, and handling their specimens. For example, many sperm banks stipulate that donors should be no older than forty, to minimize health hazards associated with aging, and have fathered no more than ten children with their donated sperm, to decrease the risk of half-sibling marriage in the future. Most sperm banks also require donors to supply personal and family medical histories and to undergo physical exams, blood typing, and psychological interviews to determine their fitness.

Once a male donor receives a clean bill of health, he can provide a sperm sample, which is then frozen, subsequently thawed, and evaluated through semen analysis. The sample must meet minimum post-thaw standards of 20 to 30 million sperm per milliliter and 25 to 40 percent motility, with normal appearance.

Acceptable sperm samples are quarantined for six months, at which time the donor must be retested for disease. If his results are negative at that point, his sperm can be donated.

Purchasing Donor Sperm

Sperm is ordered and shipped in vials. It's usually sold in one of two forms: *unwashed*, meaning it is still in the semen and is ready for insertion in the cervix, or *prewashed*, meaning it has been separated from the semen and is ready for intrauterine insemination, IVF, or other ART procedures.

Although some doctors prefer that you buy prewashed sperm, many fertility clinics recommend that patients purchase unwashed sperm because it freezes and thaws much better than prewashed sperm. Fertility clinics have the ability to do the washing just prior to the insemination procedure. Even though it's a bit more expensive to wash the sperm on-site, it's cost-effective in the long run because it takes fewer attempts to be successful. In either case, you'll likely have to order several vials.

How good is frozen sperm? In general, sperm tolerates the freezing and thawing process very well. Frozen sperm is not as viable as fresh sperm, but with today's reproductive technologies, doctors can achieve very good pregnancy rates with frozen sperm. Most samples can be held in liquid nitrogen indefinitely. In fact, if you're thinking of having another child, ordering and storing extra sperm at your doctor's office can be advantageous. Often, when a couple is ready to have another child, the donor is no longer available, so they need to select someone else. By storing excess donor sperm, however, your children can have genetic siblings.

11

Donor Eggs and Embryos

When having a baby with your own eggs or embryos isn't possible, you have another option: a donor. For some couples, using someone else's genetic material is an easy, straightforward choice. But for others, the idea of using donor eggs or embryos can challenge their values, beliefs, and attitudes. It can prompt the age-old question about what ultimately influences children: nature or nurture, heredity or environment? Yet, choosing to use donor eggs or embryos offers a woman a chance to become pregnant and carry a child.

Donor Eggs

In principle, any woman can use donor eggs. For the most part, however, women who choose this option have fertility or health issues that prevent them from becoming a mother in any other way. These issues include the following:

- *Perimenopause and postmenopause.* Advancing age is the most common reason for working with an egg donor.
- *Premature ovarian failure (POF).* Women under age forty may use an egg donor because their ovaries aren't functioning properly.
- *Genetic factors.* A woman may choose to use someone else's eggs because she carries the gene for a genetic disease or defect. She may be fertile but not want to pass along her health problem, particularly if only her gene is necessary to do so.

- *Repeated in vitro fertilization (IVF) failures.* Many women consider using donor eggs when in vitro fertilization hasn't worked for them.

Choosing an Egg Donor

Donor eggs can come from either a woman you know or a woman you don't know. If a family member or friend has volunteered to donate her eggs, you won't have to look further as long as she meets the health criteria.

Known Donors

A known donor is usually a female relative, friend, or woman you've met through an intermediary. Couples who work with someone familiar to them do so for various reasons. The biggest advantage is that you already know much about the donor. If it's your sister, for instance, you share DNA. If it's your lifelong friend, you're likely aware of her family and social history.

But there is a downside to familiarity. You need to seriously consider what it might mean to have continued, close contact with your child's genetic mother. Although there are no legal or ethical restraints on using a sister, cousin, or close friend as a donor, you need to consider the emotional risk of future interactions between your child and the donor.

Whomever you select, make sure you've done your research, especially if your egg donor is not a close relative or friend but is someone you've met through another person. Without a donor agency, you're on your own to make sure the individual meets all of the important criteria. Since Food and Drug Administration (FDA) guidelines mandate that fertility clinics fully screen all egg donors for medical and genetic diseases, as well as psychological and emotional stability, you have some protection.

Unknown Donors

In the vast majority of cases, egg donors are unrelated to the couple. Usually, it's simply easier to draw from a pool of unknown young women willing to contribute their eggs than to find someone in your circle willing to have her ovaries stimulated with medication and her eggs retrieved through needle aspiration.

Many fertility clinics recruit their own egg donors; others recommend independent agencies or brokers that specialize in finding and matching appropriate donors with couples. In either case, the clinic or agency does the initial solicitation and screening of prospective candidates. Agencies have larger donor pools than fertility clinics do; however, donor eggs purchased through fertility clinics typically cost less because the middleman fee has been eliminated.

Some fertility clinics have IVF patients who are willing to donate their excess eggs. But this option offers a fairly limited pool. You're probably better off casting your net wider. If you want to scout the entire country through the Internet, remember that your choice will have to meet your fertility specialist's approval.

In any case, unknown egg donors are usually young, in good health, and from a cross section of the general population. They represent various races, ethnicities, religions, intellects, and social and economic levels. Most are driven by altruism and empathy but also appreciate the money they're likely to earn. What else do they have in common? They arrive on the scene and quickly disappear, leaving shortly after their eggs have been retrieved.

Screening Egg Donors

Once you've narrowed your choice, your fertility specialist must ensure that your donor passes the requisite FDA testing and other medical evaluations. Until the woman's eggs are retrieved, she's actually under your doctor's care, which means your doctor is in charge.

Mandatory Testing

As with sperm donors, prospective egg donors must be screened for communicable and sexually transmitted diseases, such as human immunodeficiency virus (HIV), hepatitis B and C, Chlamydia, syphilis, and gonorrhea. They're also checked for genetic and psychological disorders. If your donor is your sister or close friend, there may be some flexibility in the timeline for the testing process. But if she's someone you've never met, she must undergo testing thirty days prior to egg retrieval.

Even if the donor's results are normal, she may still be excluded for other reasons. Something as quirky as having traveled to certain areas of the world during certain years can be a disqualifier. The FDA has a long list of countries with past and present public health issues that, if traveled to, could exclude a woman from donating her eggs. For example, if a woman was in Great Britain during the mad cow disease scare, she is automatically eliminated as a donor.

Personal/Medical History

Beyond being free of communicable diseases, egg donors must be good medical risks. Every prospective candidate must answer an exhaustive questionnaire detailing her personal, reproductive, and family medical histories. Ethical fertility clinics and donor agencies apply stringent criteria, based on national regulations and guidelines, in their screening process. For instance, all egg donors must be of legal age to provide informed consent.

Since younger women respond better to ovulation stimulation and produce more and higher-quality eggs than older women do, the traditional cutoff age for donors is early to mid-thirties. Doctors often make judgment calls on age, however, as long as the individuals involved understand the downsides, such as an increased risk of Down's syndrome when the genetic mother is older.

If a woman has donated her eggs in the past, must she be a "proven" donor? Not necessarily. Even if none of the previous recipients became pregnant, you still may have success with her eggs. What's more important is the number of times she's donated her eggs. American Society for Reproductive Medicine (ASRM) guidelines suggest that a woman donate her eggs no more than six times, to protect both donor and recipient.

Genetic screening is usually done based on the frequency of specific diseases in certain ethnicities: cystic fibrosis in Caucasians; Tay-Sachs disease in Ashkenazi Jews; and sickle-cell anemia in African-Americans. But there are limitations. Fertility clinics and donor agencies screen for the most common genetic diseases and the most frequently occurring mutations. So unless the donor's family history raises a red flag, something may be missed. Fortunately, that's rare.

Elective Criteria

Even though a woman's personal characteristics have little to do with her suitability or risk as a donor, they are often very important to a couple who is considering using her eggs. A major part of donor selection is finding someone who is an appropriate match for you and your partner. Not surprisingly, most couples gravitate toward donors who resemble the female partner. The screening questionnaire provides basic descriptions and characteristics of a donor. In addition, many clinics and agencies today provide photos, videos, and even personal statements to give couples the fullest picture possible of a donor. Unlike testing and medical information, there are no rules concerning these elective criteria.

Trusting Donor Eggs

Even with screening, can people lie? Of course they can. But everything humanly possible is done to keep donors honest. Fertility clinics, in particular, have come a long way, by regulatory force and through professional evolution, in what they require of candidates. Because the process is more structured today than it was years ago, couples can be fairly confident in the screening process as long as they're dealing with an established fertility clinic or donor agency. Although clinics and agencies must be licensed in individual states, the criteria vary, as does the diligence with which some still screen candidates.

Reputable programs follow strict ethical standards and perform comprehensive screening. Anonymous donors, in particular, must explain their motivation for donating their eggs in an initial questionnaire that includes many other personal, health, sex, and even drug questions. They also must undergo the Minnesota Multiphasic Personality Index (MMPI), a 500-question, true-false test that reveals personality traits that might not be desirable. The results are especially important for couples who believe personality is genetic. Some agencies even offer temperament screens to further understand how a prospective donor thinks and acts. Many also make counseling sessions with a mental health professional mandatory to ensure that donors are capable of consenting to the procedure, cognizant of related issues, and sincere in their intentions.

The most important step is to choose a reputable fertility clinic or donor agency that adheres to stringent standards, is very selective in its candidate choices and has many controls in place. But in the end, you'll also have to simply trust.

Donor Embryos

If either you cannot contribute eggs or your male partner cannot provide sperm, you still have another option: donated embryos—embryos created by the sperm and eggs of another couple. Often, embryos are donated by couples undergoing IVF who couldn't use their entire supply. Although some fertility clinics encourage couples to donate their excess embryos, doing so is not a universal practice. Many couples choose to discard them rather than make them available. The alternative is to seek out an agency that focuses on embryo donation or to find a fertility clinic that has a good donor embryo program.

Another option is to secure donated sperm and eggs and merge them in the laboratory. Choosing the latter means your fertility specialist will need to synchronize a larger group of people than with conventional IVF. Although the same mechanics of joining eggs and sperm outside the uterus apply, there's one difference: Instead of collecting fresh sperm from your partner, your doctor will be using sperm that has been frozen.

Whatever the source, all of the same preliminaries apply in terms of screening and testing. In the case of embryos created previously by a couple for their own use, the FDA recommends, rather than requires, donor testing. It mandates the screening, however, if the embryos are created specifically for donation. If you're the recipient, you will need to have your uterus evaluated to make certain you can carry the fetus. To ensure that your endometrium is ready for implantation, you'll also undergo estrogen and progesterone therapy prior to embryo transfer.

In the absence of universal laws explicitly dealing with embryo donation, couples contemplating using a known donor embryo may want to consult an attorney. Although there have been no cases of genetic parents reclaiming rights to their donated embryos, you want to make sure that you've completed all the necessary legal agreements cementing your parental rights to the child. With anonymous donor embryos, you'll likely have no difficulty with parental rights, since the informed consent that a donor couple signs giving up their extra embryos serves as proof that they've waived all future rights to any offspring. Also, fertility clinics are bound by both the Hippocratic oath and federal privacy Health Insurance Portability and Accountability Act (HIPAA) regulations to never divulge information about the identity of donors.

12

Gestational Carriers

If you are unable to become pregnant and carry a child, you may wish to explore the idea of having another woman carry your baby. Although this may seem like a simple concept, there are emotional, medical, and legal issues to consider. These issues depend, in part, on the type of arrangement you choose—a traditional *surrogate* or a *gestational carrier.*

Surrogate or Gestational Carrier?

If you choose to have another woman carry your baby, should you consider a traditional surrogate or a gestational carrier? What's the difference, and why is it important?

A traditional surrogate is a woman who not only carries and delivers a baby, but also donates her own eggs. She is inseminated with your male partner's sperm. A gestational carrier, however, offers only to carry the baby. The baby's parents create the embryo that is then transferred to the carrier's uterus. The carrier has no genetic link to the baby.

The use of both traditional surrogates and gestational carriers is legal in forty-four states, but illegal in six. Both forms of surrogacy are subject to strict guidelines from the FDA.

Most reputable fertility clinics don't recommend or participate in true surrogacy. Why? It presents potential problems with the surrogate mother. Because she is the genetic mother, she may have legal grounds if she decides she wants to keep the baby. No matter what she was paid or how ironclad the original contract was between her and the parents, she's still considered the birth mother.

Such legal difficulties don't exist with a gestational carrier. Because the woman is not genetically related to the baby, she has no legal claim to the child. A correctly executed contract between a couple and a gestational carrier is usually binding.

If a woman has no eggs or uterus and still wants to pursue surrogacy, she and her partner may choose to use eggs from a donor and have them implanted in the uterus of a gestational carrier. This, too, avoids any legal risks with the surrogate mother.

Choosing a Gestational Carrier

As with egg donors, a gestational carrier may be someone you know or someone you don't know and, instead, meet through an agency.

Unknown Gestational Carriers

If you choose an unknown gestational carrier, you won't have the close relationship you would likely have with a carrier you know personally. And even though you'll get to know an unknown carrier over time, she won't be an active part of your life once the delivery is over…unless you want her to be.

Since there are many gestational carrier agencies and brokers across the country, you need to select carefully. Your fertility specialist can recommend an agency or broker that's trustworthy in the way it screens potential candidates and matches them with couples. Ethical agencies have strict criteria, beginning with the age of a carrier—she should be at least twenty-one and have delivered a child at term that she's currently raising. A woman who has not had a child of her own may not be aware of the feelings she might have about a child after carrying and giving birth to him or her.

In addition to a physical examination, a candidate must be willing to undergo the same infectious disease screens that embryo and sperm donors undergo. She also must undergo an evaluation of her uterus as well as other tests for underlying conditions that might complicate the pregnancy. Not surprisingly, a common requirement is that gestational carriers be nonsmokers.

Most ethical agencies take their time screening potential carriers. During the three- to five-month selection process, a potential carrier usually undergoes counseling with a mental health professional to ensure that she fully understands what she's agreeing to do. The sessions explore issues such as managing the relationship with the intended parents, coping with her own attachment to the fetus, and handling the impact of a pregnancy on her own friends and family.

By putting the candidate through an intensive screening process, an agency not only ensures that a potential gestational carrier is comfortable with her commitment but that she also has support from her own family. The counseling process also gives professionals a chance to learn enough about a woman to make the best match to the couple.

Known Gestational Carriers

What if you wish to use a known gestational carrier—a woman you know? She could be a family member or friend who's volunteered to carry your baby. Clearly, there are advantages to this. You would be familiar with the woman's lifestyle, health habits, and even her sense of responsibility. Yet, the same warnings about engaging a known egg donor apply with a known gestational carrier.

This woman you know, who would carry your baby, would still be among your circle of family or friends after the baby is born, and she may feel emotionally linked to the child. Some women are concerned that such a link may cause uncomfortable situations in the future. For this reason, many women are more comfortable choosing a carrier they don't know. Still, if the carrier you choose is someone you know, she will be required to meet the same medical requirements as an unknown carrier and will be required to enter into a legal contract with you.

Why Women Become Gestational Carriers

A carrier's motivations for carrying another woman's baby are several. She may enjoy being pregnant and have a desire to help others. Many women have such an uncomplicated pregnancy history that it's relatively easy for them to carry a child. They're willing to be pregnant because they feel genuine empathy for another woman who can't experience the same joy. Is financial gain a motive? Yes, money is a factor, although most agencies require that a prospective carrier be financially secure. (She can't be receiving government assistance.) The carrier may want to add to her family resources, but being a carrier can't be how she earns a living.

Your Relationship with a Carrier

A gestational carrier becomes an active part of your life. She's someone you will get to know and follow during the next nine months. Many couples feel it's their duty and right to accompany the woman to her prenatal appointments, and they want to participate in labor and delivery.

A gestational carrier is also someone with whom you'll have a financial relationship. How much will her participation cost? There are few guidelines or restrictions on how much money a gestational carrier can ask for. In some states, however, the only money allowed to change hands is that needed for reasonable expenses. Your carrier may have medical insurance of her own that covers maternal services, regardless of the circumstances. But since that's not always the case, you'll likely need to pay all of her medical expenses in addition to the agency and carrier fees. These fees can include those for prenatal testing, treatment for any unexpected pregnancy-related problems, follow-up care, and maybe even a tummy tuck if the carrier has multiples.

There can be other challenges with gestational carriers. The decision-making becomes more complicated. For example, what happens if there's a risk of multiple births but opinions differ on selective reduction? Who makes the final decision?

You'll likely address many of these issues during your first discussions or counseling sessions with a carrier. As part of the process, most agencies require that intended parents and a gestational carrier meet with a mental health professional to address specific roles, expectations, and potential problems during the pregnancy. You want to arrive at a consensus on how your carrier should behave to ensure a healthy pregnancy and what you need to do to support her. It is important that you be confident that the carrier is willing to pay the same close attention to the pregnancy as you would.

In addition to details on financial terms, legal gestational carrier agreements usually include specific language as to medical interventions, embryo transfers, and selective reduction in case of multiple pregnancies or fetal anomalies. You'll also need to legally have your names affixed to the birth certificate, listing you as your baby's biological parents. States differ on how the process is handled; some allow the birth certificate to be prepared prior to delivery.

All of these issues should be part of a legal agreement. You'll need a lawyer very well schooled in third-party reproduction, so that you, your baby, and the gestational carrier are protected.

Steps to Pregnancy

Once you've engaged your gestational carrier, you and your partner can begin focusing on making a baby. In vitro fertilization (IVF) has made gestational carrier pregnancies possible. Because a woman's eggs are fertilized outside her body, the resulting embryos can be easily transferred into the uterus of another woman.

As with donor eggs, however, the challenge is to synchronize the two cycles so that the carrier's uterus is ready for the embryos created from your fresh eggs. For several weeks prior to IVF, your carrier will take estrogen to thicken her uterine lining in anticipation of the pregnancy. Several days after your eggs are retrieved and fertilized with your partner's sperm, your doctor will transfer the resulting embryos into her uterus.

Once eggs are retrieved, the process moves forward like any IVF procedure. Once the embryo has been successfully implanted, the pregnancy proceeds with careful monitoring of the progress. In most cases, the new parents are present for the delivery.

A Final Word

If you're discouraged about achieving pregnancy, don't be. Today, fertility is a recognized field of medicine that encompasses a wide range of sophisticated and diagnostic procedures and treatment options. Physicians have significantly increased their understanding of female and male infertility. With the vast array of resources now available, if you are having problems conceiving, you have treatment options. By choosing a fertility specialist and staying committed, there's a good chance you'll succeed.

Glossary

Abortion: Termination or loss of a pregnancy prior to twenty weeks gestation. Abortions can be spontaneous (miscarriage) or induced or elective (a voluntary interruption of pregnancy).

Acrosome: Area on the head of the sperm that contains enzymes that allow it to penetrate the egg.

Adhesion: Scar tissue that joins one organ to a neighbor organ; can be the result of surgery, infection or other trauma.

Age factor: Major female fertility factor for women because it relates to diminished ovarian reserve.

American Society for Reproductive Medicine (ASRM): Multidisciplinary organization that promotes quality practices in the field of infertility.

Amenorrhea: Complete absence of menstrual periods, either failure to begin menstruation by age 18 or six months of absent periods in a woman who has had previous cycles.

Anabolic steroids: Group of synthetic hormones used by athletes to increase bulk because they promote the growth and storage of tissue. Can cause problems with male fertility.

Anaphylactic shock: Widespread and serious allergic reaction that can end in death.

Anovulation: Complete absence of ovulation or release of an egg from the ovary.

Antibodies: Substances produced by the body's immune system to protect against viruses, bacteria and other foreign invaders.

Antiphospholipid antibodies: Antibodies that work against the fatty cells of the blood vessel walls and platelets; they can result in micro blood clots that cause a miscarriage.

Antigens: Foreign substances capable of producing of antibodies when introduced into the body. They include allergens, toxins, bacteria, foreign blood cells and cells of transplanted organs.

Apotosis: A natural form of programmed cell death.

Artificial Insemination: Delivering prepared sperm directly into a woman's reproductive tract via syringe and catheter to increase the odds of conception.

Asherman's syndrome: Severely scarred uterine tissue often found after a D&C procedure, elective abortion or from an IUD, making embryo implantation difficult.

Assisted hatching: Micro-manipulation procedure performed on embryos before they're transferred to the uterus with in vitro fertilization. A tiny opening is made in the zona pellucida or outer wall of the egg using a laser or special chemical to enhance the likelihood of implantation.

Assisted reproductive technology (ART): Number of treatments in which a woman's eggs are removed from the ovary, fertilized outside the body, and then transferred back into the body. The most frequently used ART procedure is in vitro fertilization or IVF.

Atresia: Process by which cells regress, die, and are subsequently reabsorbed by the body. Atresia is one of the ways a woman supply diminishes over her lifetime.

Azoospermia: Absence of sperm.

Bartholin glands: Two glands located slightly below and to the left and right opening of the vagina; secrete mucus; help lubricate the vagina.

Basal Body Temperature: Means of timing ovulation by charting a woman's temperature at rest each day. Theoretically, BBT rises after ovulation has occurred.

Bicornuate uterus: Uterus with two protruding, horn-shaped ridges that create the shape of a heart.

Biopsy: Removal of tissue sample for microscopic evaluation.

Blastocyst: Fertilized embryo after five days of development.

Blastomeres: Cells resulting from the cleavage or division of a fertilized egg during early embryonic development.

Carbon dioxide: Gas pumped into the abdominal cavity during an endoscopic procedure to expand the space, thus improving a surgeon's view of the organs.

Cautery: Removing or sealing damaged tissue by chemical or electrical means.

Centers for Disease Control and Prevention (CDC): Federal government's public health agency. Tracks fertility clinic statistics, particularly in vitro fertilization.

Cervical factor: Problems with a woman's cervix that can impede the sperm from impregnating an egg.

Cervical mucus: Lubricant secreted by the cervix to transport sperm through the canal into the uterus so it can reach the fallopian tube and fertilize the egg.

Cervical stenosis: Cervix that is so restricted or tight normal sperm passage is difficult.

Cervix: Sphincter or circular muscle at the lower part of the uterus.

Chlamydia infection (*Chlamydia trachomatis*): Most common of sexually-transmitted diseases, it causes no symptoms in 50 percent of cases but can damage the fallopian tubes and other reproductive tract organs and lead to infertility.

Chromosome: Threads of DNA in a cell's nucleus that transmit hereditary information. Each cell contains 46, with half inherited from each parent.

Clomiphene citrate (Clomid): Most common of oral fertility drugs, it's used to stimulation.

Colposcopy: Test to look at the vagina and cervix through a lighted magnifying tool or colposcope.

Cone biopsy: Extensive form of cervical biopsy so called because a cone-shaped wedge of abnormal tissue is removed from the cervix and examined under a microscope.

Corpus luteum: Remodeled structure of the follicle after the egg is released. It secretes both estrogen and progesterone and sustains the pregnancy until the placenta forms.

Cytoplasm: One of three parts of the cell, the cytoplasm contains substances important to the cell's function. The cell also contains a nucleus, which contains genetic material, and the zona pellucida, the outer coating.

Cryopreservation. Freezing sperm, eggs and embryos for future use.

Cryosurgery: Application of extreme cold to destroy abnormal tissue.

Cumulus cells: Fluffy layer surrounding an egg that is indicating that it has matured into an embryo ready for transfer.

Cyst: Abnormal sac filled with fluid.

Day 1: First day of normal menstrual flow.

DES (diethylstilbestrol): Synthetic estrogen prescribed to pregnant women during the 1950s and 60s. Some girls exposed to DES in utero experience uterine abnormalities that can affect their fertility and ability to carry a baby.

Dilation and curettage (D&C): Surgical procedure that involves dilating the cervix and scraping the lining of the uterus; often performed after a miscarriage.

Diminished ovarian reserve: Sometimes synonymous with age factor, it refers to fewer and fewer healthy, viable eggs available for conception as a woman grows older.

DNA – deoxyribonucleic acid: Genetic code or blueprint necessary to construct and direct each cell in the body.

Double uterus: Refer to the most common structural abnormality of the uterus whereby a fibrous or connective band of endometrial tissue divides the cavity, creating the potential of repeated miscarriages. Also referred to as a septate uterus.

Donor insemination: Artificial insemination with donor sperm.

Ectopic pregnancy: Pregnancy that occurs outside the uterus, most often in the fallopian tubes. Also referred to as a tubal pregnancy.

Ejaculate: Sperm, along with proteins, minerals, vitamins and other substances, that are emitted in semen during ejaculation.

Ejaculatory ducts: Male ducts that contract with orgasm to cause ejaculation.

Embryo: Fertilized egg.

Embryo transfer: Transferring laboratory-fertilized embryo to the uterus.

Embryologist: Specialist trained to do microscopic work in the laboratory with sperm, eggs, and embryos.

Endometrial biopsy: Removal of a tissue fragment from the uterine lining for microscopic study.

Endometrial polyps: Usually benign fleshy, growths that appear inside the uterus, contributing to embryo implantation problems.

Endometriomas: One kind of ovarian cyst; also referred to chocolate cysts because of the blood-thickened material they ooze when drained.

Endometriosis: Disease that occurs when cells similar to those lining the uterus implant in abnormal places such as the abdominal cavity, ovaries, and around the fallopian tubes.

Endometrium: Lining of the uterus.

Epididymis: Tightly coiled, thin-walled tube that moves sperm from the testicles to the vas deferens.

Epididymitis: Inflammation of the epididymis, which can cause scarring and blocked ducts as well as testicular swelling.

Estradiol: Most important form of naturally-occurring of the female hormone family of estrogens.

Estrogens: Female sex hormones produced by ovary that causes female characteristics and also play a role in physiology, menstruation and pregnancy.

Factor V Leiden: Inherited propensity for abnormal clotting due to a mutation of the factor that helps platelets form around an injury during healing.

Fallopian tube: Conduit between the ovaries and uterus responsible for delivering fertilized eggs to the uterus.

Fecundity: Woman's personal chances of conception in any given month.

Fertilization: Joining the egg and sperm to create an embryo.

Fibroid (Leiomyoma): Benign tumors found in the uterine muscle and connective tissue; they can prevent an embryo from implanting and growing.

Fimbria: Fingered ends of the fallopian tube that pick up the egg following ovulation and send it down the tube.

Follicle: Fluid-like sac within the ovary that contains the immature egg.

Follicular phase: Stage of the menstrual cycle from the onset of a woman's period until the egg releases (ovulation).

Follicle-stimulating hormone (FSH): Secreted by the pituitary gland, FSH causes eggs to mature in a woman each month. It also stimulates the production of sperm in men.

Gamete: Cells of reproduction; oocytes (eggs) in women and sperm in men.

Gamete intrafallopian transfer (GIFT): Assisted reproductive technology performed by placing both sperm and egg directly into a woman's fallopian tubes.

Genes: DNA segments that carry genetic information in the form of DNA.

Gestational carrier: Woman who carries and delivers another couple's baby. Differs from a traditional surrogate in that the carrier doesn't use her own eggs so she has no genetic linked to the baby. She becomes pregnant with the couple's embryo.

Gestational diabetes: Form of diabetes that occurs in pregnancy. Usually diagnosed at 28 weeks, it can surface in women who have no history of diabetes prior to pregnancy and may have no further problem after delivery.

Gonadotropin: Hormone that has a stimulating effect on the ovaries and testes. Comes from the words *gonad,* meaning a reproductive organ, and *tropin,* a hormone that stimulates another hormone.

Gonadotropin-releasing hormone (GnRH): Hormone produced by the hypothalamus that controls reproductive function by controlling the production of FSH and LH.

Gonorrhea: Sexually transmitted disease caused by the bacteria, *neisseria gonorrhoeae*; may impede fertility by damage parts of the female reproductive tract

GnRH agonists and antagonists: Medications that prevent premature LH surge and ovulation; used to help control spontaneous ovulation with IVF

Hepatitis B and C: Two of six viral infections that can cause severe liver inflammation. Can be life-threatening if passed to a growing fetus.

Higher-order multiple pregnancies: Pregnancy with three or more gestations.

Histology: Microscopic study of cells and tissue.

Hormone: Chemical produced by one gland of the endocrine system to exert its effect on another part. It travels from location to location via the bloodstream.

Hostile mucus: Cervical mucus that impedes rather than aids a sperm's progression through the cervical canal.

Human chorionic gonadotropin (hCG): Hormone produced by developing pregnancy to help the corpus luteum produce progesterone. Injectible hCG induces ovulation and progesterone production.

Human menopausal gonadotropin (hMG): Luteinizing and follicle-stimulating hormone recovered from the urine of post-menopausal women. Injectible hMG triggers ovulation.

Hyperprolactemia: Excessive prolactin in the blood.

Hyperstimulation: Enlargement of the ovaries following ovulation induction.

Hyperthyroidism: Overactive thyroid.

Hypothalamus: Area of the brain responsible for maintaining various bodily functions. It controls the hormones that regulate menstruation.

Hypothyroidism: Underactive thyroid.

Hysterosalpingogram (HSG): Sophisticated X-ray procedure that involves injecting radiopaque dye into a woman's uterus and tubes to visualize her cervix, uterus and fallopian tubes.

Hysteroscopy: Procedure in which a tiny instrument is inserted into the vagina and up into the uterus, giving a physician a panoramic view of the uterine cavity and allowing the doctor to diagnose and treat many abnormalities.

Hysteroscopic polypectomy: Procedure that uses a special lit hysteroscope threaded through the vagina to view the uterus and remove offending polyps by scraping the lining.

Immunobead test: Test performed on blood serum or seminal fluids to detect the presence of directed antibodies that could interfere with sperm transport or egg fertilization. Often used in cases of unexplained or idiopathic infertility as well as vasectomy reversal.

Immunoglobulin G (IgG): Antibodies that reflect the presence of a previous infection.

Immunoglobulin M (IgM): Antibodies that reflect the presence of a current or recent infection.

Implantation: Attachment of the embryo to the wall of the uterus.

Incompetent cervix: Weak cervix that fails to remain closed as the developing fetus grows.

Infertility: Inability to conceive after one year of unprotected intercourse or the inability to carry a pregnancy to term delivery.

Intracytoplasmic sperm injection (ICSI): Assisted reproductive technology that involves injecting a single sperm directly into the center of the egg.

Intramural fibroids: Benign growths that develop within the muscle of the uterine wall. By distorting the cavity, they can interfere with conception.

Intrauterine Insemination (IUI): Procedure in which a very thin, flexible catheter carrying washed sperm is threaded through the cervix and into the uterus where it's delivered.

In vitro fertilization (IVF): Assisted reproductive technology that involves removing a woman's mature eggs, fertilizing them outside her body, and then transferring the embryos to her uterus for implantation.

Klinefelter's syndrome: Abnormality in which an extra X chromosome on a man's XY complement of chromosomes can result in decreased testicle size and sperm counts.

Kruger Morphology Strict Criteria: Standards by which embryologists analyze and select sperm, particularly prior to in vitro fertilization. Widely accepted as the best predictor of male fertility potential.

Laparoscope: Fiberoptic scope inserted through the naval that gives doctor a panoramic view of the reproductive organs.

Laparosocopy: Surgical procedure in which the reproductive organs are visualized, evaluated, and corrected via a special scope threaded through the navel.

Loop electrosurgical excision procedure (LEEP): Use of thin, low-voltage electrical wire to cut out abnormal cervical tissue revealed during a colposcopy, a special magnified examination of the cervix.

Lupus antioagulants: Antiphospholipid antibodies that can cause small blood clots in the placenta, which impede nutrition to a growing fetus, resulting in miscarriage.

Luteal phase: Second half of the menstrual cycle — the two weeks after ovulation when the lining of the uterus readies itself for implantation of the embryo.

Luteinizing hormone (LH): Pituitary hormone responsible for inducing the release of a mature egg from its follicle.

Male factor infertility: Infertility involving the man's reproductive system.

Meiosis: Normal cellular division that eventually results in a mature egg ready to be fertilized.

Menopause: Cessation of menstruation for at least one year, on average around age 51, after which a woman is no longer able to become pregnant.

Menstrual cycle: Monthly cycle of hormone production and ovarian activity that either prepares the body for pregnancy or produces menses (the period). The cycle starts on day one of the period.

Methylenetetrahydrofolate reductase (MTHFR): Cellular enzyme that can raise other chemicals, called homocysteines, leading to pregnancy-ending high blood pressure.

Microscopic Epididymal Sperm Aspiration (MESA):
Retrieval method whereby the sperm is removed from the epididymis through a small percutaneous or skin incision.

Micro-manipulation: Process by which eggs and embryos are manipulated in the laboratory using instruments under a microscope. Used specifically in ICSI and assisted hatching.

Minnesota Multiphasic Personality Index (MMPI): Most frequently used of all personality tests, the MMPI involves 500-plus true-false questions designed to determine personality traits and propensity for depression or other serious mental health issues.

Miscarriage: Loss of a fetus.

Multiple-gestation pregnancy: Pregnancy that includes more than one fetus.

Mullerian ducts: Ducts that develop into parts of the female reproductive system.

Obstetrician-gynecologist (OB-GYN): Specialist in the female reproductive system.

Oligospermia: Decreased number of sperm.

Oocyte: Female egg.

Ovaries: Two robin-egg-sized organs that produce the egg and female sex hormones.

Ovarian cyst: Noncancerous, fluid-filled sac located in or on the ovary that can be a normal component of the ovulatory cycle.

Ovarian failure: Complete loss of ovarian function.

Ovarian Hyperstimulation Syndrome (OHSS):
Complication that develops when the ovaries are overstimulated during the use of fertility medications. The ovaries enlarge and cause a build-up of fluid in the abdominal cavity. Symptoms include sudden weight gain, abdominal pain, nausea, vomiting, and low urine output. In rare cases, ovarian hyperstimulation can result in death.

Ovulation: Release of the egg from the ovary.

Ovulation induction: Use of medications and/or hormones to induce multiple eggs to develop.

Ovulatory Factor: Most common female fertility factor; involves interruption of a woman's normal ability to produce healthy eggs.

Pelvic adhesions: Fibrous bands that form between and around organs preventing them from functioning normally.

Pelvic inflammatory disease (PID): Inflammation and scarring of the pelvic region caused by untreated sexually transmitted diseases and pelvic infections.

Percutaneous Epididymal Sperm Aspiration (PESA): Technique of removing sperm by penetrating the scrotal skin with a needle and drawing a small amount of sperm from the epididymis. It's the least used of all retrieval methods.

Peri-menopause: Ten years or so leading up to menopause, during which time a woman's egg supply diminishes significantly.

Peritoneal factor: Fertility problems that originate with the peritoneum, the tissue sheath that covers your abdominal cavity. The most common example is endometriosis.

Pipette: Narrow, calibrated tube, usually glass, into which small amounts of liquid are suctioned for measurement or transfer.

Pituitary gland: Small gland within the brain responsible for regulating hormones associated with many aspects of metabolism, fluid balance, milk production and the menstrual cycle.

Placenta: Organ that develops within the uterus during pregnancy to provide the fetus with nourishment and eliminate waste products. It also produces hormones necessary to sustain the pregnancy.

Polar body: Cellular fragment spun off during the process of meiosis or division indicating an egg is mature and ready for fertilization.

Polycystic ovary syndrome (PCOS): Frequent cause of irregular or absent menstrual periods caused by hormonal imbalances. Its name refers to the presence of small cysts that form on the ovaries.

Polyploidy: Three or more sets of chromosomes inside each cell indicating a problem with the embryo. Sperm and egg begin as *haploid,* meaning they each carry half or 23 of the 46 chromosomes necessary to create a new embryo in their *pronuclei.* The normal merging of the two creates a single, *diploid* nucleus containing 23 chromosomes from each contributor. Because polyploidy indicates the presence of extra chromosomes, it also signals that the embryo won't survive. The presence of polyploidy is a red flag in grading embryos for transfer.

Postcoital test: Test to evaluate the interaction of the sperm and the cervical mucus.

Preeclampsia: Pregnancy-induced high blood pressure. Also known as toxemia.

Preimplantation genetic diagnosis (PGD): Genetic test that involves removing a single cell or blastomere from an embryo to test for chromosome abnormalities or single gene mutations prior to implantation.

Premature ovarian failure (POF): Loss of ovarian function before age 40.

Progesterone: Steroid hormone in females produced mainly in the second half of the cycle by the corpus luteum in the ovary and placenta. It prepares the uterus for implantation.

Prolactin: Pituitary hormone responsible in part for breast milk production.

Proliferative phase: The follicular cycle of a woman's menstrual cycle, named for the thickening of the endometrium.

Pronuclei: Refers to the centers of an individual sperm and egg. During fertilization they merge into a single *diploid* nucleus, which contains the 46 chromosomes necessary to create a new embryo, 23 from each pronuclei.

Prostatitis: Inflammation of the prostrate resulting in testicle swelling and other symptoms.

Recombinant DNA technology: Culturing a portion of human DNA that controls FSH production in the laboratory to manufacture almost pure FSH

Reproductive endocrinologist: Ob-gyn who has completed a three-year fellowship in reproductive endocrinology, including training in infertility and reproductive medicine.

Retrograde ejaculation: Condition in which the semen is thrust backward into the bladder rather than discharging from the penis upon ejaculation.

Reversal of sterilization: Reconnecting fallopian tubes that have been tied, cut or burned using microsurgical techniques.

Rubella: German measles. Loss of immunity as a woman ages can result in birth defects if she contracts the condition during the first trimester of her pregnancy.

Secondary infertility: Inability to conceive after previously having carried a pregnancy to viability.

Secretory phase: Part of the uterine cycle that corresponds to the luteal phase. During this part of the cycle the endometrium prepares for pregnancy.

Selective reduction: Multi-embryo fetal pregnancy reduction performed to lessen pregnancy and pre-maturity risks.

Septate uterus: Most common structural abnormality of the uterus whereby a fibrous or connective band of endometrial tissue divides the cavity, creating the potential of repeated miscarriages. Also sometimes referred to in lay terms as a double uterus.

Septum: Abnormal tissue barrier separating the cavity of the uterus.

Semen analysis: Laboratory evaluation of sperm sample to determine its viability to impregnate egg. Criteria include semen volume plus sperm count, movement and shape.

Sertoli cell-only syndrome: Rare genetic condition in which sperm producing cells, called Sertoli cells, in the testicles never form during fetal development.

Sexually-transmitted diseases: Bacterial infections transmitted through sexual conduct. Conditions such as Chlamydia, gonorrhea, and syphilis can impede fertility.

Single gene mutation: Change or mutation on a apart or sequence of a single gene resulting in more than 300 disorders.

Society for Assisted Reproductive Technology (SART):
Primary organization of professionals who practice
assisted reproductive technologies (ART), including in
vitro fertilization.

Speculum: Instrument inserted in the vagina and opened to
allow visualization of the cervix.

Sperm: Male gamete; each contain a male's genetic material.

Sperm motility: Movement of sperm.

Sperm morphology: Sperm shape.

Sperm count: Number of sperm in the ejaculate.

Sperm donation: Use of man's sperm that has been donated
for either an artificial insemination or IVF procedure.

Sperm motility: Motion of the sperm.

Spermatic cords: Cord-like structure in males formed by the
vas deferens and arteries, veins, nerves, lymphatic vessels
and other tissue. It's surrounded by several layers of
connective tissue, which protect the contents. Passing
down from the abdomen to each testicle, the two cords
act as conduits for semen.

Subcutaneous: Under the skin.

Submucosal fibroids: Benign growths in the uterine wall
lining that push into the uterine cavity, making it too
small to carry a developing fetus.

Surrogacy: One woman carrying a pregnancy for another
woman. A traditional surrogate has a genetic link to the
child because she donates her own eggs. A gestational
carrier, however, carries the embryo of another couple
and has no genetic connection.

Syphilis: Sexually transmitted disease caused by bacteria,
treponema pallidum.

Testicle: Male organ that produces sperm and male sex
hormones.

Testicular biopsy: Procedure performed to determine if the
cells that produce sperm in the testicles are present.

Testicular Sperm Extraction/Aspiration (TESE/TESA):
Involves removing small tissue samples from the
sperm-rich tube at the back of the testis for eventual
extraction of sperm.

Testosterone: Principle male sex hormone responsible for male characteristics.

Thyroid gland: Endocrine gland in front of the neck that produces hormones that regulate the body's metabolism.

Toxemia: Pregnancy-induced high blood pressure. Also known as preeclampsia.

Traditional surrogate: Woman who offers her eggs and uterus to childless couples. Because of a genetic link to the child, surrogates are a less desirable way to have a child than a gestational carrier, who is free of any genetic links to the baby.

T-shaped uterus: Abnormally long, narrow and underdeveloped uterus formed in a woman as a result of being exposed in utero or in the womb to *diethylstilbestrol* or *DES*, a synthetic estrogen given to her mother during pregnancy. Prescribed during the 1940s to the 1960s, DES caused various birth defects and other problems in babies, including the t-shaped uterus.

Tubal factor: Disorders of the fallopian tubes that prevent conception.

Tubal ligation: Surgical sterilization of a woman by tying the fallopian tubes.

Tubal pregnancy: Pregnancy outside the uterus, most often in the fallopian tubes. Also referred to as an ectopic pregnancy.

Ultrasound: Use of high-frequency sound waves to view internal reproductive organs. Transvaginal refers to positioning the transducer or wand inside the vagina versus moving it over the abdomen.

Unexplained infertility: Diagnosis given when a couple is inexplicably unable to conceive (see "infertility") in spite of a completed, normal evaluation.

Unicornuate uterus: Uterus shaped like the horn of a unicorn; it's half the size of a normal uterus.

Urethritis: Inflammation of the urethra, the tubing that carries sperm, semen and urine through the penis.

Urologist: Specialist in the urinary tract of both sexes and often in male reproduction.

Uterine factor: Infertility caused by growths or other anomalies in the uterus that prevents an embryo from implanting and developing.

Uterine septum: Excess tissue wall partially or totally dividing the uterine cavity.

Uterus: Female reproductive organ in which an egg is implanted and pregnancy develops.

Varicoceles: Varicose or dilated veins in the scrotum.

Variococelectomy: Surgery to repair a varicocele, or varicose vein of the scrotum.

Varicella: Chicken pox. Loss of immunity as a woman ages can result in birth defects if she contracts the condition during the first trimester of her pregnancy.

Vas deferens: Tubes through which sperm and testicular fluid move to the ejaculatory ducts.

Vasectomy: Surgical sterilization of a man by interrupting both vas deferens, which prevents the sperm from reaching the ejaculate.

Vitrification: Rapid as opposed to slow freezing of eggs or embryos to ensure quality.

Washed sperm: Sperm separated from semen ad other toxins for safe injection into the uterus.

World Health Organization (WHO) standards: Guidelines for measuring sperm quality and potential for fertility.

Zona pellucida: Protective coating surrounding the embryo.

Zygote: Egg that has been fertilized but has not yet begun to divide.

Zygote intrafallopian transfer (ZIFT): Procedure that involves fertilizing eggs in the laboratory and then inserting the resulting zygotes into a woman's fallopian tube.

Resources

American College of Obstetricians and Gynecologists (ACOG)
PO Box 96920
Washington DC 20090-6920
(202) 638-5577
www.acog.org

Professional organization representing 52,000 OB-GYNS. Offers locator service as well as information on all female obstetric and gynecological problems, including topics affecting fertility.

American Fertility Association
315 Madison Ave., Suite 901
New York, NY 10017
(888) 917-3777
www.theafa.org

Leading consumer source of fertility information. Offers monthly newsletter, "Ask the Expert" online feature, monthly "webinars," toll-free-support line, plus physician, therapist, and other professional resources.

American Society for Reproductive Medicine (ASRM)
1209 Montgomery Highway
Birmingham, AL 35216-2809
(205) 978-5000
www.asrm.org

Nonprofit organization devoted to advancing knowledge and expertise in reproductive medicine. Beyond establishing guidelines for fertility programs, ASRM provides comprehensive information on all aspects of diagnosis and treatment.

American Urological Association Foundation

1000 Linthicum Blvd.
Linthicum, MD 21090
(800) 689-3800
www.UrologyHealth.org

Professional organization dedicated to specialists who treat urinary tract problems of men and women. Site offers information on infertility as well as directory of urologists.

Centers for Disease Control and Prevention (CDC)

1600 Clifton Rd.
Atlanta, GA 30333
(404) 639-3311
www.cdc.gov/reproductivhealth/index.htm

Federal reporting agency. Reports success rates on assisted reproductive technology as well as publications on various related topics.

Endometriosis Association

8585 N. 76th Place
Milwaukee, WI 53223
(800) 992-3636
www.endometriosisassn.com

Self-help organization devoted to empowering and educating women about this puzzling disease. Web site includes information on endometriosis as well as other resources.

International Council on Infertility Information Dissemination (INCIID)

P.O. Box 6836
Arlington, VA 22206
(703) 379-9178
www.inciid.org

Consumer-based infertility organization launched by women facing the problem. INCIID emphasizes the importance of seeking quality care early through consumer-targeted information about the latest cutting-edge technology, discussion forums, and newsletters. It also offers a professional service roster.

Polycystic Ovarian Syndrome Association (PCOSA)
PO Box 3403
Englewood, CO 80111
www.pcosupport.org

PCOSA seeks to raise awareness of polycystic ovarian syndrome through education, newsletter, support network and other services. Provides links to other organizations.

RESOLVE: The National Infertility Association
1760 Old Meadow Rd., Suite 500
McLean, VA 22102
(703) 556-7172
www.resolve.org

Offers a wide variety of resources including fertility information, adoption and related topics plus local chapter and support groups listings and links to professionals.

Society for Assisted Reproductive Technology (SART)
1209 Montgomery Highway
Birmingham, AL 35216-2809
(205) 978-5018
www.sart.org

Organization dedicated to professionals who work in assisted reproductive technologies. Offers a wide variety of information for patients including individual IVF program success rates. Affiliate of ASRM.

The Society of Reproductive Surgeons (SRS)
1209 Montgomery Highway
Birmingham, AL 35216-2809
(205) 978-5000
www.reprodsurgery.org

Professional organization of ASRM members with special interest and competency in reproductive surgery. Promotes excellence in gynecologic and urologic reproductive surgery through education, professional development and research.

Index

A

abortions, 21, 28
absent periods, 42
adrenal gland, 17, 31
age-related diminished
    ovarian reserve, 32
alcohol use, 2, 83, 84
American Association of
    Tissue Banks (AATB), 95
American Society for
    Reproductive Medicine
    (ASRM), 58, 95, 101
amino acid, 39
amniocentesis, 60
amniotic fluid, 60
anabotic steroids, 76, 80, 82
aneuploidy, 60
anger, 5
anovulatory, 16
Antagon, 45, 47
antibiotics, 80
antidepressants, 80–82
antifungals, 80
antihypertensives, 80, 82
antiphospholipid antibodies
    (APAs), 36–38
antisperm antibodies
    (ASAs), 24, 36, 39, 40, 78,
    79, 90
appendix, 19

acquired immune
    deficiency syndrome
    (AIDS), 95
Asherman's syndrome, 21
assisted hatching, 56, 57
assisted reproductive
    technologies (ARTs),
    49–67, 96
azoospermia, 76

B

bacterial infections, 19
Bartholin glands, 13
basal body temperature
    (BBT), 40
benign tumors, 69
bicornuate uterus, 22, 70
biochemical pregnancy
    biochemical, 66
birth defects, 23, 60
bladder, 73
    repair, 82
blastocyst, 55
    transfer, 56
bleeding
    abnormal, 21
blood clots, 46
blood estradiol test, 53
blood hormone levels, 27
blood testing, 36–40, 82, 83
blood thinner, 38

130

body temperature, 40, 41
Bravelle, 45
breast milk production, 17, 30, 31
Brown, Louise, 49

C

causes of infertility, 1, 2, 16–25
Centers for Disease Control and Prevention (CDC), 65
cerebral palsy, 58
cervical mucus, 24, 39, 49, 74
   reduction, 43
cervical problems, 23, 24
cervical stenosis, 23
cervix, 2, 12–14, 23, 32, 33, 50
   damage, 49
cetrorelix acetate, 47
Cetrotide, 45, 47
chicken pox, 36, 95
Chlamydia, 2, 19, 20, 36, 51, 77, 100
chocolate cysts, 25
choosing a physician, 26, 27
chorionic villus sampling (CVS), 60
chromosomal disorders, 76
chromosomal testing, 78
chromosome 21, 60
chromosome abnormalities, 60, 61
chromosome disorders, 79
chromosomes, 60
clinical pregnancy, 67
Clomid, 42, 45
clomiphene citrate, 42, 43, 45, 89
   side effects, 43

congenital disorders, 79, 80, 82, 92
controlled ovarian overstimulation, 43
coping emotionally, 4–11
coping skills, 5–7
corpus cavernosum, 73
corpus luteum, 16, 32, 46
corpus spongiosum, 73
corticosteroids, 90
costs for treatment, 3
Coumadin, 38
Crinone, 45
cryopreservation, 63–65
cystic fibrosis (CF), 61, 80, 101
cytomegalovirus (CMV), 95

D

day 3 estradiol test, 30, 32
day 3 folliclel-stimulating hormone (FSH) testing, 32
day 3 luteinizing hormone (LH) testing, 32
deep venous thrombosis, 37, 38
denial, 4, 5
depression, 5, 80
diabetes, 81
diagnosing infertility, 26–41
diethylstilbestrol (DES), 23
dilation and curettage (D & C), 21
DNA (deoxyribonucleic acid), 60, 74, 99
donor eggs, 3, 98–104
   choosing a donor, 99, 100
   genetic testing, 101
   known, 99
   legal agreements, 104
   medical history, 101

recruitment, 100
unknown, 99, 100
donor embryos, 98–104
donor insemination, 92
donor sperm, 79, 92–97
   purchasing, 96, 97
Down's syndrome, 60, 61
ductal system, 83
   blockage, 80, 81, 91
   damage, 90, 91

E

early embryo stage, 55
ectopic pregnancy, 20, 23,
   36
egg, eggs, 30, 43
   dominant, 16
   donation, 51, 98–104
   examination, 53
   fertilization, 54, 55
   frozen, freezing, 64
   maturation, 52, 53
   preparation, 53
   removal, 51, 69
   retrieval, 53
   see also donor eggs
egg donors, 98–104
   mandatory testing, 100,
     101
   screening, 100–103
egg production, 2, 32, 43,
   50
egg reserve, 30
ejaculation, 73, 81
   retrograde, 81
ejaculation malfunctions, 76
ejaculatory ducts, 81
electrolyte replacement, 46
embrologist, 88
embryo, 16, 31, 34, 36, 54,
   61
   determining sex, 62
   development, 53

donation, 62, 98–104
frozen, 52, 57
frozen, freezing, 64, 65
genetic testing, 60–62
transfer, 55, 66, 109
embryologist, 55, 57, 61
emotional boundaries, 10
emotional support, 4–11
ending treatment, 11
endocrine problems, 83
endocrine system, 14
endometrial biopsy, 32, 33
endometrial polyps, 21
endometrial tissue
   removal, 69
Endometrin, 45
endometriomas, 25
endometriosis, 3, 24, 25, 28,
   69
   lesions, 35
endometrium, 13–15, 32,
   48, 50
environmental toxins, 83
epididymis, 73, 80, 87, 88
   inflammation, 77
epididymitis, 77
erectile dysfunction, 74
erection or ejaculation
   problems, 49, 73, 74, 80,
    81
estradiol, 2, 30–32, 53
estrogen, 12, 16, 31, 104
   deficiency, 18
exercise, 6
   excessive, 17

F

factor V Leiden, 38
fallopian tubes, 2, 12, 14,
   16, 25, 33, 34, 50, 74
   blockage, 19, 34
   damage, 36
   infections, 24

problems, 19, 20
scarring, 19, 20
treatment, 35, 71
family history, 29
family support, 9, 10
female hormones, 31
female infertility, 12–25
 causes, 16–25
female reproductive system,
 12–16
fertility clinic, 7, 102, 103
 choosing, 65–67
fertility drugs, 3, 42–48, 89
 side effects, 43
fertility evaluations, 8
fertility specialist, 3, 27,
 100, 103
fertility treatment
 procedures, 49–67
fertilization, 12
fetus, 13, 30, 38, 48
fibroid tumors, 3, 20, 33,
 35, 69, 70
follicles, 14, 15, 32, 33
 monitoring, 40
follicle-stimulating hormone
 (FSH), 14–16, 31, 32, 44,
 45, 50, 57, 74, 83
 Higher-than-normal
  levels, 79
 low levels, 78
follicular menstrual cycle
 phase, 15
Follistim, 45
Food and Drug
 Administration (FDA), 51,
 64, 65, 93, 95, 99–101,
 103, 105–110

G

gamete intrafallopian tube
 transfer (GIFT), 57, 59,
 69

ganirelex acetate, 47
gene, genes, 60
gene mutations, 36, 60
genetic abnormalities, 60
genetic code, 60
genetic disorders, 92
genetic factors, 98
genetic testing, 60–62, 80
German measles, 36, 95
gestational carrier, 3,
 105–110
 choosing, 106, 107
 financial relationship,
  108
 known, 107
 legal agreements, 109
 legal issues, 105, 106
 motivation, 107, 108
 relationship with, 108,
  109
 screening, 106
 unknown, 106
glans, 73
gonadotropin-releasing
 hormone (GnRH), 14, 31,
 69
gonadotropin-releasing
 hormone (GnRH)
 agonists, 47
gonadotropin-releasing
 hormone (GnRH)
 antagonists, 47
Gonal-F, 45
gonorrhea, 100
guilt and blame, 5
gynecologic examination,
 29
gynecologic history, 28
gynecologist, 82

H

Health Insurance Portability and Accountability Act (HIPAA), 104
heart disease, 81
heavy menstrual bleeding, 20
hemophilia, 61
heparin, 38
hepatitis, 36, 37, 51, 95, 100
hernia repair, 82
high blood pressure, 39, 46, 58, 80, 81
higher-order multiple births, 62, 63
high-order multiple births, 58
Hippocratic oath, 104
homocysteine, 39
hormone, hormones, 2, 12–14, 16, 17, 83
  deficiencies in men, 77, 78
  evaluation, 29–32
  imbalances, 76, 89, 90
hormone imbalances, 2
hostile cervical mucus, 24
human chorionic gonadotropin (hCG), 16, 31, 45, 53, 76, 80, 82, 89
human immunodeficiency virus (HIV), 51, 95, 100
human menopausal gonadotropin (hMG), 44, 45, 50, 89
  side effects, 44
hyperthyroidism, 29
hypogonadotropic hypogonadism, 78
hypothalamus, 13, 14, 30, 31
hypothyroidism, 29

hysterectomy, 69, 70
hysteroscopy, 35, 69, 70

I

idiopathic condition, 76
immune system, 78
immunological disorders, 76, 78, 79, 90
impotence, 81
in vitro fertilization (IVF), 3, 44, 46, 48, 51–55, 57, 64, 68, 79, 80, 88–91, 96, 103, 109
  failures, 57
  repeated failures, 98
inducing follicle development, 52, 53
infections, 76, 77, 83
infertility
  causes, 1, 2, 16–25
  diagnosing, 26–41
  treatment options, 2, 3
  types, 2
inflammation of the testicles, 77
injectable gonadotropins, 43–47, 52
insulin levels, 17
insulin-altering drugs, 18
insurance issues, 3
intercourse, 73, 75, 81, 90
intracytoplasmic sperm injection (ICSI), 54, 57, 64, 80
intramural fibroids, 21
intrauterine insemination (IUI), 39, 40, 44, 46, 49–51, 57, 84, 89–91, 96
irregular periods, 42

K

kidney failure, 46
kidneys, 82

Klinefelter's syndrome, 79
Kruger, Thinus F., 84
Kruger's Strict Morphology, 84, 86

L

laparascopy, 35, 68, 69
laparotomy, 70
leuprolide acetate, 47, 69
Leydig cells, 74, 78
lifestyle factors, 2
liver, 37
low body weight, 17
low-dose prednisone, 40
Lupron, 45, 47, 69
lupus anticoagulants, 36, 38
luteal menstrual cycle
    phase, 16, 17, 30, 48
luteal phase defect, 30, 33
luteinizing hormone (LH),
    14–16, 31, 32, 41, 44, 53,
    74, 83
    higher-than-normal
        levels, 79
    low levels, 78

M

male hormones, 74
male infertility, 1, 72–86
    causes, 75–81
    diagnosing, 81–86
    treatment, 87–91
male reproductive organs,
    73, 82
    damage, 92
medical history, 17, 19,
    27–29, 82
medications that affect
    sperm count, 76, 80, 82
meditation, 7
menopause, 15, 29, 43
Menopur, 44, 45

menstrual cycle, 13, 16,
    28–30
    irregularities, 17
    phases, 15, 16
menstrual disorders, 32
methotrexate, 20
methylenetetrahydrofolate
    reductase (MTHFR)
    deficiency, 39
microadenomas, 30
micro-clotting, 55
microsurgery, 70, 71, 91
microsurgical epididymal
    sperm aspiration (MESA),
    87, 88
    advantages, 88
Minnesota Multiphasic
    Personality Index
    (MMPI), 103
miscarriage, 21, 28, 30, 33,
    37, 67
    prevention, 55
motile sperm, 51, 75, 88, 90
multiple births, 44, 51, 67
    prevention, 58, 59
mumps, 77
mycoplasma, 51

N

nervous system, 14
nicotine, 2, 83
Novarel, 45

O

obesity, 17
obstetric history, 28
obstetrician-gynecologist
    (OB-GYN), 26
occupational toxins, 83
oligo-ovulatory, 17
oligospermia, 76
oral progestin, 42
orchitis, 77

ovarian hyperstimulation
syndrome (OHSS), 44,
64, 65
complications, 46, 47
ovarian reserve, 18
ovarina follicles
see follicles
ovary, ovaries, 12, 14, 30,
31, 33, 43, 50, 51, 69
cysts, 17, 25, 35, 69
enlarged, 46
hyperstimulation, 52
infections, 24
polyps, 33–35
removal, 28
treatment, 35
overactive thyroid, 29
Ovidrel, 45
ovulation, 2, 30
prevention, 47
ovulation induction, 50
ovulation problems, 1
ovulation stimulation, 101
ovulation-predictor kits
(OPKs), 40
ovulatory menstrual cycle
phase, 15
ovulatory problems, 16–18,
43

P

Pap smear, 32
partner support, 7, 8
pelvic adhesions, 19, 24, 69
pelvic inflammatory disease
(PID), 19, 21
pelvic pain, 20
pelvic ultrasound, 17, 18,
33
penis, 73, 74, 77, 83
percutaneous epididymal
sperm aspiration (PESA),
88

performance anxiety, 81
Pergonal, 44, 45
perinatologist, 62
peritoneal problems, 24, 25
peritoneum, 24
physical examination, 29,
82
pituitary gland, 14, 17,
29–32, 44, 78
pituitary tumors, 30
placenta, 31, 38, 60
polycystic ovarian
syndrome (PCOS), 17, 18
diagnosing, 17
polyps
see ovary, ovaries
potassium chloride, 62
prednisone, 55, 79, 90
preeclampsia, 39, 58
pregnancy
clinical, 67
types, 66
pregnancy rates, 71, 89, 90
Pregnyl, 45
preimenopause, 98
preimplantation genetic
diagnosis (PGD), 60, 61
premature delivery, 38, 58,
63
premature ovarian failure
(POF), 17, 18, 32, 64, 98
preterm labor, 23
previous pregnancies, 28
primary care physician, 82
primary infertility, 2
prior vasectomy, 80
progesterone, 12, 16, 30,
31, 45, 55, 104
deficiencies, 30
supplemental, 48
prolactin, 17, 31
testing, 30

prolactinomas, 30
proliferative menstrual
cycle phase, 15
Prometrium, 45
pronuclei, 54
prostate gland, 73, 74, 80,
83
inflammation, 77
surgery, 81
prostatic fluids, 73
prostatitis, 77
Provera, 42
pseudoephedrine, 91
psychological issues, 81
puberty, 15
pubic bone, 73

R

recreational drugs, 2, 83, 84
repeated in vitro
fertilization (IVF) failures,
98
reproductive
endocrinologist (RE), 26,
27, 68, 82
reproductive
endocrinology, 26
reproductive history, 58
reproductive organ
evaluation, 33–35
reproductive surgery, 68–71
procedures, 68–71
Repronex, 44, 45
RESOLVE (National
Infertility Association), 6
retrograde ejaculation, 81,
91
retroverted uterus, 22
rubella, 95
see German measles

S

saline-infusion
sonohysterography (SIS),
33
scrotal veins, 76
scrotum, 72, 78, 83, 88
secondary infertility, 2
selective reduction, 62, 63
semen, 51, 74
evaluation, 84
liquefaction, 85
morphology, 83
motility, 83
viscosity, 85
volume, 76, 83, 84
semen analysis, 79, 82–86
seminal fluids, 80, 81
seminal vesicles, 73, 74
seminiferious tubules, 72
septate uterus, 22, 70
Serophene, 42, 45
Sertoli cell-only syndrome,
79
serum progesterone test, 30
sex linked disorders, 61
sexual response, 14
sexually transmitted
diseases (STDs), 2, 19,
24, 95, 100
sickle-cell anemia, 61, 102
single gene mutation, 60,
61
smoking, 2
Society for Assisted
Reproductive Technology
(SART), 65, 66
sonohysterogram (SHG), 33
sperm, 39, 40, 43, 72–86
analysis, 82
appearance, 75, 85
collection, 54, 83, 84
concentration, 85

decreased, 76
density, 85
donation, 51, 92–97
evaluation, 84
frozen, freezing, 63, 88, 96, 97
function, 85
harvesting, 87–89
morphology, 75, 85, 86
motile, 51
motility, 75, 85, 88, 90
nonmotile, 90
parts, 74
prewashed, 96
problems, 75, 76, 87–91
quality and quantity, 2, 49
storage, 97
washed, 51, 63, 96
zero, 89
sperm bank, 88, 94
licensure, 95
sperm count, 8, 27, 49, 83
decreased, 75
volume, 76
zero, 76
sperm donor, 92–97
choosing, 93, 94
known, 93
screening, 94–96
testing, 95
unknown, 93
sperm parameters, 75
sperm production, 2, 7, 72–86, 90
decreased, 78
spermatic cords, 89
spinal cord defects, 39, 81
steroids, 55, 84
stress, 17
stress management, 6, 7
subfertile, 87
submuscosal fibroids, 21

success rates, 55, 66
Sudafed, 91
superficial thrombosis, 38
supplements that affect sperm count, 76
support groups, 6
surgeon
choosing, 68
syphilis, 51, 95, 100

T

Tay-Sachs disease, 61, 102
testcular sperm aspiration (TESA), 88
testicles, testes, 72, 73, 83
shrinkage, 79, 80
trauma, 82
testicular biopsy, 88, 89
testicular problems, 83
testicular swelling, 77
testosterone, 74, 78–80, 82, 89
thyroid gland, 17, 29
thyroid hormones, 29
thyroid problems, 2
thyroid-stimulating hormone (TSH), 29, 31
thyroxin (T4), 29, 31
timed intercourse, 44, 46, 49
tobacco use, 2
transducer, 33
transvaginal ultrasound, 33, 50
treatment options, 2, 3
triiodothyronine (T3), 29, 31
triplet births, 62
Trisomy 21, 60
t-shaped uterus, 23
tubal ligation, 28
reversal, 71
tubal pregnancy, 69

type 2 diabetes, 17
types of infertility, 2

U

ultrasound, 53, 55, 80
underactive thyroid, 29
undescended testicle, 79
unexplained infertility, 25, 49
unicornuate uterus, 23
urethra, 73, 78
  inflammation, 77
urethral swab culture, 77
urethritis, 77
urinary tract, 81, 82
urologist, 81, 87, 89–91
uterine abnormalities, 69
uterine fibroids, 20
uterine fluid, 56
uterine lining, 22, 30, 31, 43, 48
uterine problems, 20, 21
uterine septum, 22
uterine wall, 56
uterus, 2–14, 16, 22, 32, 33, 50
  removal, 69
  treatment, 35

V

vagina, 12, 13, 14, 50, 74
varicella
  see chicken pox
varicoceles, 76, 77, 82, 83
  treatment, 89
varicose veins of the
  testicles, 76
vas deferens, 73, 80, 88, 91
vasectomy, 78, 80, 82, 88, 91
  reversal, 78, 90
vitrification, 64, 65
vulva, 13

W

warfarin, 38
washed sperm, 59, 63
  see also sperm
World Health Organization
  (WHO) standards, 84, 86

X

x-linked disorders, 61

Y

y chromosome abnormality, 79
yoga, 7

Z

zygote intrafallopian tube
  transfer (ZIFT), 57, 59, 69

About the Authors

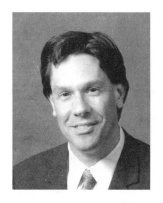

Gerard M. Honoré, Ph.D., M.D., is a founder of Perinatal and Fertility Specialists of San Antonio, Texas, a comprehensive fertility care center with a highly successful in vitro fertilization (IVF) program. He also specializes in advanced assisted reproductive technologies (ARTs), as well as surgery for endometriosis, polycystic ovarian syndrome (PCOS), and other infertility-related problems.

Dr. Honoré earned his Ph.D. from Duke University, Durham, North Carolina, and his M.D. from Wake Forest University, Winston-Salem, North Carolina, where he also completed a residency in obstetrics and gynecology (OB/GYN). He then completed a reproductive endocrinology and infertility fellowship at the University of Texas Health Science Center, San Antonio, where he later served as assistant professor of reproductive endocrinology.

Dr. Honoré has authored more than thirty scientific articles, abstracts, and book chapters on reproductive medicine. Certified by the American Board of Obstetrics and Gynecology, he is a Fellow of the American Congress of Obstetricians and Gynecologists and is a member of numerous professional organizations dedicated to reproductive medicine. He's been named often as one of America's "Top Obstetricians and Gynecologists" and as one of the "Super Doctors" in Texas.

Visit Dr. Honoré at **www.pfspecialists.org**.

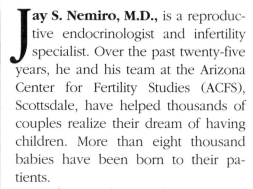

Jay S. Nemiro, M.D.,** is a reproductive endocrinologist and infertility specialist. Over the past twenty-five years, he and his team at the Arizona Center for Fertility Studies (ACFS), Scottsdale, have helped thousands of couples realize their dream of having children. More than eight thousand babies have been born to their patients.

After graduating from medical school and completing an obstetrics and gynecology residency at George Washington University, Washington, D.C., Dr. Nemiro completed a fellowship in reproductive endocrinology and infertility at Georgetown University, also in Washington, D.C. Dr. Nemiro founded ACFS in 1982, with a commitment to the successful evaluation and treatment of infertility and to the emotional well-being of couples and individuals facing the challenges of infertility. Since then, he's been at the forefront of reproductive medicine research and technology.

The author of many peer-reviewed articles on infertility, Dr. Nemiro has lectured extensively on the subject. For many years, he served as director of reproductive endocrinology and infertility in the Department of Obstetrics and Gynecology at Good Samaritan Hospital, Phoenix, Arizona, where he trained hundreds of OB/GYN residents, receiving multiple teaching awards. Dr. Nemiro has also been featured as an authority in reproductive medicine in numerous national publications and television interviews.

Visit Dr. Nemiro at **www.acfs2000.com**.

Consumer Health Titles from Addicus Books
Visit our online catalog at www.AddicusBooks.com

After Mastectomy—Healing Physically and Emotionally . . . $19.95

Bariatric Plastic Surgery $24.95

Body Contouring after Weight Loss $24.95

Cancers of the Mouth and Throat—
A Patient's Guide to Treatment $14.95

Cataract Surgery $19.95

Colon & Rectal Cancer—
A Patient's Guide to Treatment $14.95

Coronary Heart Disease—
A Guide to Diagnosis and Treatment $15.95

Countdown to Baby $19.95

The Courtin Concept—Six Keys to Great Skin at Any Age . . . $19.95

The Diabetes Handbook—Living with Type II Diabetes $19.95

Elder Care Made Easier $16.95

Exercising through Your Pregnancy $19.95

Facial Feminization Surgery $49.95

The Healing Touch—Keeping the Doctor/Patient
Relationship Alive under Managed Care $9.95

LASIK—A Guide to Laser Vision Correction $19.95

Living with P.C.O.S.—Polycystic Ovarian Syndrome,
2nd Edition $19.95

Look Out Cancer Here I Come $19.95

Lung Cancer—A Guide to Treatment & Diagnosis $14.95

The Macular Degeneration Source Book $14.95

The New Fibromyalgia Remedy $19.95

The Non-Surgical Facelift Book—
A Guide to Facial Rejuvenation Procedures $19.95

Overcoming Infertility $19.95

Overcoming Metabolic Syndrome $19.95

Overcoming Postpartum Depression and Anxiety $14.95

Overcoming Prescription Drug Addiction $19.95

Overcoming Urinary Incontinence $19.95

A Patient's Guide to Dental Implants $14.95

Prostate Cancer—A Patient's Guide to Treatment $14.95

Sex and the Heart $19.95

A Simple Guide to Thyroid Disorders $19.95

Straight Talk about Breast Cancer—
   From Diagnosis to Recovery *$19.95*
The Stroke Recovery Book—
   A Guide for Patients and Families *$19.95*
The Surgery Handbook—
   A Guide to Understanding Your Operation. *$14.95*
Understanding Lumpectomy—
   A Treatment Guide for Breast Cancer *$19.95*
Understanding Parkinson's Disease, 2nd Edition *$19.95*
Understanding Peyronie's Disease. *$16.95*
Understanding Your Living Will. *$12.95*
Your Complete Guide to Breast
   Augmentation & Body Contouring *$21.95*
Your Complete Guide to Breast Reduction & Breast Lifts . . . *$21.95*
Your Complete Guide to Facial Cosmetic Surgery *$19.95*
Your Complete Guide to Facelifts *$21.95*
Your Complete Guide to Nose Reshaping *$21.95*

To Order Books:

- **Visit us online at:** www.addicusbooks.com
- **Call toll free:** 800-352-2873

For discounts on bulk purchases, call our Special Sales Dept. at (402) 330-7493